COUNSELING THE AGING AND THEIR FAMILIES

Edited by Irene Deitch, PhD
& Candace Ward Howell, MS

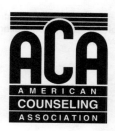

AMERICAN
COUNSELING
ASSOCIATION

■ ■ ■

THE FAMILY PSYCHOLOGY AND COUNSELING SERIES

Jon Carlson, Editor

Counseling the Aging and Their Families

10 9 8 7 6 5 4 3 2 1

American Counseling Association
5999 Stevenson Avenue
Alexandria, VA 22304

Director of Acquisitions
Carolyn Baker

Director of Publishing Systems
Michael Comlish

Cover design by Martha Woolsey

Library of Congress Cataloging-in-Publication Data

Counseling the aging and their families / edited by Irene Deitch &
   Candace Ward Howell.
       p.   cm.
   Includes bibliographical references.
   ISBN 1-55620-163-X (alk. paper)

       1. Aged—Counseling of. 2. Aged—Family relationships.
   3. Caregivers—Counseling of. 4. Family counseling. I. Deitch,
   Irene. II. Howell, Candace Ward.
   HV1451.C63   1996
   362.6'6—dc21   96-48067
                                                              CIP

The Family Psychology and Counseling Series

Counseling the Aging and Their Families
Irene Deitch, PhD and Candace Ward Howell, MS

Counseling Families with Chronic Illness
Susan McDaniel, PhD

Mid-Life Divorce Counseling
Lita Linzer Schwartz, PhD

Transitioning from Individual to Family Counseling
Charles Huber, PhD

Understanding Stepfamilies: Implications for Assessment and Treatment
Debra Huntley, PhD

In Preparation

Social Construction in Couples Counseling
James Robert Bitter, EdD; Don Bubenzer, PhD, and John West

Advisory Board

■ ■ ■

THE FAMILY PSYCHOLOGY AND COUNSELING SERIES

Table of Contents

PART II. AGING AND FAMILIES: CONFLICTS AND CRISES

PART III. AGING AND FAMILIES: TRANSITION AND TRAUMA

From the Series Editor

As I read through this monograph, it became very clear to me that there is a significant change occurring in the family landscape generally and in me specifically. I realize that I am getting older. My hair is gray, I have turned 50, I have an AARP card in my wallet, and a few months ago I joined the ranks of grandparenthood. Can all of this really be true? I have noticed I am not quite as agile as I used to be. I have to think about mobility and transportation. Money and retirement are concerns that absorb more of my time with each day. My support system diminishes as parents, siblings, and friends pass away or move to warmer climates. Perhaps the most upsetting for me is their loss, as well as accepting the diminution of physical and mental prowess. Though I believe that there is more wisdom in my thoughts, I also believe I do not work quite as well as I used to. Jonathan Swift's observation that "Every man deserves to live long, but no man would be old" seems to match my own thoughts. As Oscar Wilde said, "The tragedy of old age is not that one is old, but that one is no longer young."

The population of older people is growing significantly. Life expectancy has also increased, resulting in more people living longer. As anyone who watches the *Today* show knows, it is no longer a rarity for people to celebrate their 100th birthday or their 60th wedding anniversary. It used to be that people would die at an early age and there were one, two, or at most three living generations in any one family, but now many families comprise four or five generations. The problems associated with aging pose unique challenges for counselors, and we have often been at a loss regarding how to deal with them.

In this volume, editors Deitch and Howell have brought together the leading thinkers in the field of aging and gerontology to address the implications for families and counselors. This monograph helps us to realize that most aging people remain connected to their families and that they really do have support systems. Despite what the popular press states, families make great efforts to stay together and to take care of their own.

Whether or not we really like it, we are getting old together. The capacity for growth and development is lifelong. To remain healthy as family members age, families also need to change. This volume shows us how to age in a more satisfying way.

—Jon Carlson, PsyD, EdD
Series Editor

Preface

During the past century, average life expectancy has increased dramatically, resulting in a steadily growing population of older Americans. Whereas people once succumbed to disease or illness in their 50s and 60s, advances in both prevention and treatment have made it possible for many to anticipate living 10, 20, or more years beyond the arbitrary retirement age of 65. How do these added years affect the aging and their families?

Typically the literature on family counseling has ignored the aging and their concerns (Van Amburg, Barber, & Zimmerman, 1996). Training programs for family counselors often emphasize child and adolescent development, ignoring the years on the other end of the spectrum. This monograph presents an overview of those issues that family counselors need to be aware of and trained to address in their work with the aging. The editors have drawn on the expertise of professionals in the fields of family counseling and gerontology to discuss critical developmental and clinical issues of the aging.

In chapter 1, Troll draws on research data to discuss the crucial role of aging family members as "kinkeepers" in maintaining the ongoing existence of family ties. Belsky (chapter 2) describes the demographic and socioeconomic changes that have created a generation "in the middle"—caretakers for both their children and parents—and how counselors can support them. Litwin (chapter 3) discusses the changing role of single older women in the family. Nurse (chapter 4) presents the unique challenges of families headed by older parents.

Part II looks at common points of conflict and crisis in relationships of the aging with family members. Strauss (chapter 5) describes the effect that being a grandparent has had on her, both professionally and personally. Using case material, Brok (chapter 6) illustrates the later-life developmental task of transforming the "parent–child" relationship to that of "adult–adult offspring." Brooks (chapter 7) discusses how fathers become estranged from their families and how counselors can help these men reconnect with them. Deitch (chapter 8) provides information on elder abuse, "the hidden shame of the American family."

Part III examines times of transition and trauma for families of the aging. Ronch and Crispi (chapter 9) discuss the effects of Alzheimer's disease on family members and present intervention strategies tailored to their unique needs. Through a case study, Weiner (chapter 10) describes her work with a couple affected by dementia and offers strategies for helping all family members lead satisfying lives. Saul (chapter 11) depicts the often traumatic experience of placing an aging family member in a nursing home. Finally, Doka (chapter 12) explores from a developmental perspective the loss of a parent.

It is our hope that this book will increase family counselors' awareness of common concerns of the aging, provide useful information for their work with the aging and their families, and challenge family counselors to become more "aging-friendly."

—Irene Deitch, PhD
Candace Ward Howell, MS
Editors

Reference

Van Amburg, S. M., Barber, C. E., & Zimmerman, T. S. (1996). Aging and family therapy: Prevalence of aging issues and later family life concerns in marital and family therapy literature (1986–1993). *Journal of Marital and Family Therapy, 22*(2), 195–203.

Biographies

I rene Deitch, PhD, is Professor of Psychology at The College of Staten Island, CUNY, and chairperson of Options, College Study Program for the Older Adult. She has a professional practice as a psychotherapist. Dr. Deitch is a New York state licensed psychologist and a certified family therapist and grief counselor. She specializes in issues of later adulthood and couple and family therapy. Her papers on domestic violence and mistreatment of elders are presented internationally. She has published several chapters in books on feminist psychology and the issues surrounding the elderly and their families.

She is currently a fellow of the Division of Adult Development and Aging of the American Psychological Association (APA) and president of APA's Division 46 (Media Psychology). Dr. Deitch serves on the Board of Directors for the Division of Family Psychology.

C andace Ward Howell, MS, is a counselor at the Lake Geneva Wellness Clinic, Lake Geneva, Wisconsin. She has served as associate editor of *Individual Psychology: The Journal of Adlerian Theory, Research, and Practice* and production assistant of the *Family Psychologist*. She is currently assistant editor for The Family Psychology and Counseling Series and associate editor and book review column editor of *The Family Journal: Counseling and Therapy for Couples and Families*. She has received service awards from the North American Society of Adlerian Psychology and the International Association of Marriage and Family Counselors. Ms. Howell and her husband Ken have been married for 22 years and have two children.

J on Carlson, PsyD, EdD, is Distinguished Professor at Governors State University in University Park, Illinois, and director of the Lake Geneva (Wisconsin) Wellness Clinic. Dr. Carlson has served as the president of the International Association of Marriage and Family Counselors. He has authored 20 books and over 100 professional articles including *Family Therapy: Ensuring Treatment Efficacy* (Brooks/Cole, 1997) and *The Disordered Couple* (Brunner/Mazel, 1997). He served as the editor of *Individual Psychology: The Journal of Adlerian Theory, Research, and Practice,* for 18 years. He was the founding editor of *The Family Journal.* He holds a diplomate in Family Psychology from the American Board of Professional Psychology. He is a Fellow of the American Psychological Association, a clinical member of AAMFT, and a certified sex therapist by AASECT. He has received awards for his professional contributions from the American Counseling Association, American Psychological Association, North American Society of Adlerian Psychology, and the International Association of Marriage and Family Counselors. Dr. Carlson and his wife of 29 years, Laura, are the parents of five children and grandparents of one.

Contributors

Janet Belsky, PhD, is an Associate Professor of Psychology at Middle Tennessee State University. She is the author of several books in gerontology and adult development, most recently the college text, *Adulthood in America* (West Educational Publishers, 1997).

Albert J. Brok, PhD, is director of group and couples therapy and codirector of training for the program in psychotherapy with the Generations of the Holocaust and related groups, at the Training Institute for Mental Health in New York City. He is affiliated with various postdoctoral programs and is in private practice specializing in individual, group, and couples therapy. His research interests and writings on the life cycle span a 20-year history.

Gary R. Brooks, PhD, is Acting Chief, Psychology Service, at the Central Texas Veterans Health Care System. He is an Associate Professor in Psychiatry at Texas A&M Health Sciences Center and Adjunct Faculty with Texas Women's University.

Esther Loring Crispi, PhD, a developmental psychologist, is a research associate with LifeSpan DevelopMental Systems, an interdisciplinary mental health practice and consulting group based in Poughkeepsie, New York.

Kenneth J. Doka, PhD, is Professor of Gerontology at the Graduate School of the College of New Rochelle, New Rochelle, New York.

Dorothy Litwin, PhD, is in private practice in New York City and Westchester County, New York.

A. Rodney Nurse, PhD, is in the independent practice of family and forensic psychology in Orinda, California, and the San Francisco Bay area. He is a Diplomate in Clinical Psychology (ABPP). Formerly the President of the California Graduate School of Family Psychology, he serves as a member of the Board of Directors of Rosebridge Graduate School of Integrative Psychology.

Judah L. Ronch, PhD, a clinical geropsychologist, is President of LifeSpan DevelopMental Systems, an interdisciplinary mental health practice and consulting group based in Poughkeepsie, New York. He has provided psychological services in nursing homes since 1975.

Shura Saul, EdD, BCD CSW, is a consultant in gerontological training and education as well as in family services. She is adjunct professor at a number of college and university programs in the New York area and teaches in the training programs for Long Term Care Ombudsman in Westchester and Rockland Counties. She also has a private practice in geriatrics and family counseling.

Helen M. Strauss, PhD, is Adjunct Associate Faculty at the Seton Hall University Graduate Program in Clinical Psychology, Field Supervisor at the Rutgers University Graduate Program in Applied and Professional Psychology, Faculty at the New Jersey Institute for Psychoanalysis and Psychotherapy, and Lecturer in Options: College Study Program for Older Adults. She conducts a private practice in psychotherapy and psychoanalysis in West Orange, New Jersey.

Lillian E. Troll, PhD, is Professor Emerita, Psychology, Rutgers University, and Adjunct Professor of Human Development and Aging and Medical Anthropology, University of California, San Francisco.

Marcella Bakur Weiner, EdD, PhD, is an Adjunct Professor of Psychology at Marymount Manhattan College in New York City. A Fellow of the American Psychological Association, she maintains a private practice in Brooklyn and Manhattan.

AGING: DEMOGRAPHIC AND DEVELOPMENTAL ISSUES

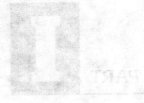

Growing Old in Families

Lillian E. Troll, PhD

There is abundant evidence that family ties have remained important in our society despite changes in family patterns and despite politically motivated declarations to the contrary (Blieszner & Bedford, 1996; Troll, 1986). The importance of these ties to individuals, however, can fluctuate over the course of a lifetime. They are perhaps less important during adolescence and more important in the relatively short years of childrearing. Bedford (1989), for example, found that even sibling relations were more important to men and women in the process of raising their children than they were to men and women in the "empty nest" period. Family ties seem to become important again as people grow old, particularly after the age of 85 (Troll, 1994). The present chapter discusses the family relations of the very old, both in terms of what old members do for their families and what families do for their old members. It also considers what the lack of such ties can mean in late life.

Gender is a significant factor in family ties at any age, and never more than in old age. Family relations of old men differ markedly from those of old women because men have usually married younger women and because women's life expectancy is longer than men's. Thus old men are more likely than old women to have a spouse living. Johnson and Troll (1992, p. S-66) noted that "gender differences in longevity result in only 44 men for 100 women at 85 years and older." Only 8% of the women in their sample of noninstitutionalized oldest-old were currently married, but 48% of the men were. The households of old men consist primarily of their wives; few old men live alone. More old women live alone in single-person households. Old women's families thus consist primarily of their children and grandchildren.

In cultures like ours, where independence is a dominant value, joint residence of parents and children commonly ends after the younger generation is grown. Only married (or cohabiting) couples and their subadult children are expected to live together. It is not surprising, then, that repeated surveys since the groundbreaking work of Ethel Shanas and her colleagues (Shanas, Townsend, Wedderburn, Fries, Milhhoj, & Stehouver, 1968) have found that old people in Western societies prefer to—and do—live apart from their children. On the other hand, they prefer to—and do—live near them. Separate residence does not mean separation from family relations. Thus the families discussed in this chapter are not necessarily people who live together; three-generation households are rare in the Western world. The families of the old are what Litwak (1960) called "modified-extended families": separate households joined together by structural and functional links.

Except for the 20% of the oldest-old who are in institutions, this trend for separate residence has been increasing. Half the men and over half the women in Johnson's (1994) sample of people over the age of 85 lived alone, even though most had notable problems managing their daily living. In addition to the value placed on independence, those who are very old today have fewer children than did their counterparts in 1900 (Treas, 1977), although there is no clear relation between number of children and residential patterns.

The present chapter deals with issues of later-life family contact and assistance as well as with feelings. It draws specifically from two sets of family data, viewing them in the light of general gerontological family literature (Blieszner & Bedford, 1996; Johnson & Troll, 1992; Troll, 1986, 1994; Troll & Bengtson, 1992; Troll, Miller, & Atchley, 1979). These data are largely intergenerational rather than intragenerational, particularly for women, since at very old ages survivors experience a progressive loss of spouses and siblings (Johnson & Troll, 1992). The differences between the two sets of data highlight the effects of health and vigor, of gender, and of availability of relatives.

The first set of data comes from a long-term study at the University of Southern California (USC). In 1971, Bengtson and his colleagues (e.g., Bengtson & Roberts, 1991) sent questionnaires to over 350 three-generation families of adults. Their primary interest then was to study intergenerational attitudes and relationships over time. The mean age of the grandchildren at the beginning of the research was 19 years. Over 2,000 individuals responded to their first mailing. There have been more than six waves of survey data collection in the 25 years since then, as well as extensive personal interviews with different subsamples. The grandparents on whom we focus in this study resided in the Los Angeles area, and most of their descendants still do. Previous analyses had focused on dyadic intergenerational comparisons. My interest was in looking at the families as units or systems.

My first reading, in 1989, of the USC files was motivated by my interest in the effect of the deaths of the grandparents on their children and grandchildren. I had been invited to use these data for this purpose and had therefore selected those families where both grandparents had died over the course of the research. In 1988, when I began, both grandparents were gone in only 11 of the families. The 10 families who agreed to participate, however, included over 100 individuals living in 30 nuclear family units or households. In addition to reading their accumulated questionnaire responses, my assistants and I interviewed several members of both the second and third generations—the survivors—in each family. As I read through the material, my interest widened from the topic of bereavement to the structure and function of these modified-extended families, particularly from the perspective of the oldest generation.

While I was working on this study, I was also collaborating with Colleen Johnson and her colleagues at the University of California, San Francisco (UCSF). In 1988, Johnson's team, (Johnson 1994) started intensive face-to-face interviewing of 150 White community residents over the age of 85, 39 men and 111 women. The primary focus in this study had been on what kinds of adaptation of very old men and women make it possible for them to live independently. Those who survived were reinterviewed at six 14-month intervals. At the end of the study, all survivors—about a third of the original sample—were in their late 90s. (A comparable sample of African American people over 85 has also been interviewed twice, but present comments are based only on the original White sample). It has been rewarding to compare the findings from these two studies.

Caretaking: Instrumental and Expressive Support

There are two sides to the family relations of old North Americans: what their families do for them and what they do for their families. Most of the gerontological literature deals with the first side—what families do for their aging members—and its focus has been primarily on instrumental services like transportation, cleaning, shopping, feeding, and nursing. We have long known that most caregiving (about 80%) to needy old people does come from their families (Johnson & Catalano, 1981; Shanas, 1979). For those who are married, spouses tend to be the primary caregivers of the needy aged—more by wives for husbands than by husbands for wives. Children usually do not step in unless a spouse in unavailable, and care by more distant relatives or friends is uncommon.

In the beginning of the San Francisco study, most of the respondents said that they did not need any instrumental help. Because they had been selected from voting records and the criterion of inclusion in the study was mental competence and community residence, they did not represent, at least in the beginning, those who were mentally incompetent or living in institutions. Many of those who did need some help, furthermore, preferred to hire people for such tasks or to get it from outside agencies rather than from their children. Consistent with the value of independence in this cohort is the belief that one should not burden one's children. In spite of this belief, however, 60% of the women at Time 1 who had children—two thirds of the sample—were getting at least some "instrumental support" from their children (Johnson & Troll, 1992). Only 30% of the men reported getting this kind of help from their children.

These figures are higher than those reported in other studies (Kovar, 1986), which showed that fewer than 20% of people who are over 70, living alone, and impaired in activities of daily living, got help from a child. Children are more likely to serve as mediators between their parents and formal service agencies, while spouses would be more likely to be the direct caregivers. Even wives who are feeble themselves take it for granted that they should take care of their husbands. One 98-year-old women said wearily that she was waiting for her 101-year-old husband to die so that she could be absolved of her responsibility and be able to die too. Besides gender differences in survival, another explanation for the gender differences in the caregiving found in the UCSF study is that the men were less disabled than the women. Apparently, those men who manage to last this long are the hardy ones.

Similar findings about family involvement were found in the Los Angeles study. The first grandparent to die in 8 of the 10 families had been taken care of by his or her spouse while the second to die was largely taken care of by their children. In 1 of the 2 remaining families, the grandparents had divorced in middle age, and in the other, where the grandparents were Italian immigrants, the grandfather had left his wife's care to their teenage daughter. In at least two of these families, grandchildren were also deeply involved with the grandparents. In one case, a college student came more than once a week to take care of his grandmother's house and garden, to shop for her, and to take her out. In another, two granddaughters—cousins—shared many parts of the final caretaking of their grandmother with their mothers. Both women had lived with these grandparents in childhood while their mothers were in the process of divorce.

But although the rendering of instrumental support has been well documented, it is what has been called "expressive support" that is the most salient contribution of family members in both these studies. In the first round of interviews in the San Francisco study, 80% of the women and 74% of the men mentioned visits, letters, phone calls, gifts, and other attentions that were meaningful to them. Of those with children, 69% of the women and 48% of the men saw a child at least weekly. Even when children lived too far away for frequent visits there were phone calls, in many families almost daily.

The importance of family ties was demonstrated by photographs displayed prominently on tables and walls. This was equally true for those whose children were no longer living—one third of the respondents in the UCSF sample had lost a child. Stories about recent family gatherings attested to the importance of such events in both studies. Golden wedding anniversaries and 90th birthday parties were almost ritual occasions. Letters and phone calls, particularly at holidays and birthdays, maintained a sense of belonging. Other research has also found that close family feelings and meaningful relationships do not necessarily demand geographic proximity (Johnson, 1993; Troll & Bengtson, 1979). It should be noted, however, that even though children are important to old people in a number of ways, few use their children as confidants or sounding boards when they are troubled. Not only does this cohort, born at the turn of the century, prefer to live and function independently, but it does not readily confide intimate details to others.

Family-Embedded versus Family-Deprived

But what about those old respondents who have neither living spouse nor children? A comparison of those in the UCSF study who might be called "family-embedded" with those who might be called "family-deprived" highlights the contrast between these two extreme groups (Troll, 1994). Previous literature on the importance of children to older people did not generally show that children contribute to a high quality of life for post-childrearing North Americans (Glenn & McLanahan, 1982). At best, parents over 65 have been found to be no happier than non-parents of the same age. Study after study (Johnson & Troll, 1994) shows that good morale in old age is associated more with having friends than with having children. It is only in advanced old age, like over 85, when friends are likely to be dead or disabled themselves, that the advantage of children becomes notable.

The children in the UCSF study provided not only instrumental and expressive help but also, significantly, linkage to the outside world. This "outside world" included other family members as well as friends. One 93-year-old woman who had no children is an example of the family-deprived group—those who had no interactions with relatives. "On Mother's Day," she said, "I sat here from 12 o'clock on and nobody came. What's so hard in taking your old aunt out with you to dinner?" While the son of her sister, whom she had taken care of from 1968 until her recent death, showed his gratitude for this service by leasing her his mother's apartment, he gave her no personal attention. In fact, by the time of the second interview, he had moved her to an institution where she remained until her death 4 years later, when she was 96. She mentioned her nephew's infrequent visits in every interview.

None of the family-deprived group was currently married and none had a child living nearby. Although 1 had a grandchild, 6 had nieces and nephews, and 1 had a surviving sibling, few of these were regular sources of help. Ten of the 17 in this group, or 59%, had no available family members at all to call on for help or companionship.

At the other end of the spectrum, all 18 family-embedded respondents had at least one child living nearby. In fact, what stands out about them is their multiplicity of relatives. In contrast to the woman described above whose only living relative was an indifferent nephew, a 90-year-old widow in the family-embedded group was deeply involved with her surviving son and particularly her daughter-in-law, from whom she heard every day. She talked about the big 90th birthday party they had given her and said that she routinely stayed with them on holidays. Through her son and daughter-in-law, she kept in touch with her grandchildren, nephews, and a long list of friends. There was little change in her health or living conditions at Time 4, when she was still close to her daughter-in-law and her oldest grandchild.

Were these two groups once the same? Were those who were now family deprived once family-embedded but had lost their connections, either through deaths or enfeeblement? This does not seem to be true. Family connectedness in the UCSF study did not change significantly from Time 1 to Time 3. Further, the family-deprived were no more disabled than the family-embedded. The difference was in their family stuctures. All of the embedded people had been married at one time, while four of the deprived had never married. Of those who needed help in the sample as a whole, 61% had some family members available. Of those with children, 77% also had other family members available but only 21% of those who had no children had such sources of help available. Or, to look at it another way, three quarters of both women and men who had children received some care, either instrumental or expressive, from their families. Some gerontologists think that having more children ensures a greater possibility of having one of them serve as a caretaker, but Uhlenberg and Cooney (1990) found that the major difference lay between having only one child or having more than one child. Having two or more children increases the chances of being family-embedded.

One interesting finding in the UCSF caregiving data (Johnson & Troll, 1992) is the rarity of substitute helpers. Shanas and her colleagues (1968) had earlier described families as "reservoirs" of helpers, with auxiliary members like nieces and grandchildren substituting for missing spouses and children. In the UCSF family data, however, the same individuals remained the chief providers of care and attention over the successive waves of interviews, even though some of the caregivers would have liked more contribution from other family members. One daugher at Time 1, for example, wished that her brother or sister would take over the responsibilities because she was about to retire and wanted to travel and feel free. Her mother had recently come to live with her. Five years later, however, she was still the only one taking care of her mother, even though her mother's health had deteriorated markedly. The only change over this period of time had been that this daughter had sought psychotherapy to help her deal with her frustration, and it did indeed make her situation more bearable. She had been the one "elected" to undertake the care of her mother because she was not married. Both her brother and sister could plead involvement with their "families."

Family Structure

The issue of size of family, mentioned above, brings us to the wider issue of family structure in general. This was a focus of my University of Southern California study, where I looked at the relative integration or organization of modified-extended families. The descendants of the 10 original sets of grandparents—three and four generations deep—did indeed exhibit systemic organization, although some of these family systems were more integrated than others. At one extreme the members met frequently for ritual holiday or birthday gatherings or phoned or dropped in for day-to-day catching up on the news and getting advice. At the other extreme the members barely knew where the others lived and had not seen each other for years.

Several explanations have been given for these differences, like family size, geographic nearness, marital stability, and gender preponderance. Smaller families are obviously easier to integrate than larger ones, and the second-most integrated family system of the 10 did indeed have the fewest members, a son and daughter in the second generation, 3 third-generation granddaughters, and only 2 great-grandchildren. But this factor did not account for much of the difference. In the most integrated family, there were 3 children and 7 grandchildren, and in one of the least integrated, there were only 2 children and 5 grandchildren.

It is true that it is easier to visit and render instrumental services when parents and children live within a block or 10 minutes' drive. But proximity is not closely related even to instrumental help. Among the UCSF respondents, some sons and daughters drove an hour to take their mother shopping or to see a doctor, while a daughter who lived in an upstairs apartment looked in on her mother in only a perfunctory way as she went off to work. One daughter in the Los Angeles study drove over half an hour at least once a week to clean her mother's house and mow her lawn and another drove 400 miles whenever her mother was sick. Besides, expressions of love or interest can be conveyed by telephone or letters and many of the 90-year-olds in the UCSF study lived for weeks on the warmth from a birthday celebration or holiday get-together.

The families in both studies live in today's society and almost all had experienced divorce. Where second marriages were stable, as in the second-most integrated family in the USC study, relations in the extended family did not seem to be affected by the marital breakup. In the least integrated family, however, the fact that both grandparents had been married several times, one of their daughters three times, and the other twice could be an important reason for their dispersion and separateness. Or maybe the underlying pathology that had influenced this lack of stability prevented their being able to stay connected.

Family Integration: Kinkeeping

It became clear that the people who had been actively responsible for most of the family organization of the 10 Los Angeles families had been the grandparents, who could be called "kinkeepers" (Rosenthal, 1985). Kinkeepers spread the family news among siblings, children, and grandchildren. They organize ritual occasions like holidays, birthdays, and weekend dinners. They monitor family needs and relationships and, when they are healthy enough, they help at times of illness or other crises. When they are not strong enough to come themselves, they arrange for other family members to help. I have written earlier (Troll, 1983) about kinkeepers' functions of monitoring family situations and jumping into the breach when necessary, of being the "family watchdogs."

But what about when the kinkeepers die or become too enfeebled to carry on their functions? At the time I interviewed the USC families, all the original kinkeeping grandparents had died, yet all the families still had a kinkeeper. These kinkeepers were now primarily the second-generation daughters who had taken over their mothers' role—or in two cases their fathers'. The transmission of kinkeeping from one generation to the next is related both to the aging process and to the process of family integration. In the USC families, the grandparents were younger than the over 85ers in the UCSF study. They continued their kinkeeping until near the end of their lives. Few San Francisco grandparents, however, appeared to have been kinkeeping for a long time. Interviewers often remarked on their apparent passivity. Even though they were still living, they seemed content to let their children become the kinkeepers for their families, which included them.

The transmission of the kinkeeping role in the USC data could be observed in the successive questionnaires. Daughters, daughters-in-law, and granddaughters were gradually becoming involved in arranging holiday and birthday gatherings. They could be said to be "in training" for the job of kinkeeping. First they assisted their mother or grandmother, then they took over the role themselves. Eventually, the location of family gatherings moved from the grandparents' homes to those of the second-generation members. Children were now more likely to pick up their parents and drive them to their own homes for celebrations, even though a good number of the grandparents' homes could have accommodated large parties.

Another factor in kinkeeping and family integration is gender. Eight of the 10 USC kinkeepers were women. In the two families where the role was performed by a grandfather, this seemed to be by default. In one of these cases, the grandmother had died young and the grandfather's second wife was the same age as his daughters. Apparently, the daughters had not yet been "trained" in kinkeeping by their mother, while the stepmother, an outsider to the family, was more involved in raising her own young children from her previous marriage than in attending to her new husband's family. Thus the grandfather had to be the one to retain contact with his widespread family; only one daughter lived near him in San Diego, two in the San Francisco Bay area, and one in the Midwest. When he died, his daughter in San Diego was nominated the kinkeeper by her sisters, but she did not seem to take the same kind of active role as the daughters in the other families. These four sisters seemed to be gradually moving apart and separating into four different modified-extended families restricted to their own children and grandchildren.

In the other male-kinkeeper family, the grandparents had divorced when they—and their children—were young, and the grandmother had led a very irregular life therafter, in and out of mental hospitals and marriages. In this case, it is interesting that the person who took over the grandfather's mantle of kinkeeping when he died was a grandson. It is yet to be seen how effectively he can reunite his siblings and their mother with the next generation, but this is his stated goal. It has long been noted that women tend to be more affiliative than are men (Troll & Bengtson, 1979).

Since in many ways gender differences are prominent in family relationships throughout life, we might expect these differences to persist into old age. And indeed, the statistics cited earlier (Johnson & Troll, 1992) do show that men are more likely to still be living with a spouse, while women are more likely to be living alone; that men are more likely to be involved with their wives while women are more involved with their children and grandchildren; and that men are more likely to be taken care of by their wives while women are more likely to be taken care of by a child. Yet when we look at larger family connections, gender differences are only relative. They become matters of whether it is men or women who keep the family together, rather than whether it is kept together at all. In the San Francisco study, there were about equal numbers of men and women among the family-embedded and among the family-deprived, for instance. Wives connect men to their larger family systems, and sons and daughters connect women to their larger family systems, but in both cases, such connections are maintained.

Just like Bernard (1973) reported for younger couples, the men in the UCSF study were more satisfied with their marriages than were the women, yet being married was not necessarily related to either good mood or perceived good health. In the USC study, about the same percentage of perceived closeness was reported for mother–daughter as for mother–son dyads (78% for each), and for father–daughter and father–son (60% versus 50%). In agreement with other family literature (Troll, 1986), mothers' relations to both sons and daughters were stronger than those of fathers. Finally, it was mostly the men who felt they had gotten closer to their grandchildren over time (50% compared with 13% of the women), closing the earlier gender difference in involvement with grandchildren. This shift could be related to the weakening of the wives' activities in family interactions rather than to a strengthening of the men's ties. Alternatively, the grandchildren might be in a better position to pay attention to their grandparents now that the fourth generation were adults, freeing the grandchildren from the demands of their own childrearing (many of the grandchildren were in their 40s and had children in their 20s.)

Generic versus Particularistic Relationships

A comparison of relations with children and those with grandchildren in the San Francisco study suggests an interesting difference between dyadic ties to particular individuals and generic ties to the family as a system. In their study of father–infant relationships, Lamb and Lamb (1976) reported that while women seemed to be linked to their families by particularistic dyadic ties, men seemed to be linked to the family as a whole. This distinction could be applied to the family relations of old people, or for that matter to family relationships in general. Both Aldous (1987) and Bedford (1992) have looked at one aspect of particularistic relationships, that of favorites among children. Aldous (1985), for example, found that parents did more for children they felt to be more needy, particularly for those who were divorced and had children. Respondents in both the USC and UCSF studies spoke more often and more fondly about some children and some grandchildren than about others. They described their children with much more particularity, by name, and their grandchildren more generically, as "my son's daughter" or "my oldest granddaughter."

Conclusion

By putting together information from the two studies described, it is possible to see the importance of family in the lives of old Americans, the way they both benefit from and contribute to their families, and the transition from active kinkeeping to being passive recipients of such kinkeeping. First, it is clear that coresidence is far from a requirement for family connectedness. Imbued with the Western value of independence, most of the old respondents studied lived by themselves if they were not currently married, and many tried to avoid "burdening" their children. The kind of help they received from either spouse or child, therefore, went beyond instrumental services to feelings of belonging and being loved, and to being connected to other family members and the world at large. Younger grandparents are the ones who keep their families integrated, who gradually "train" their children and sometimes their grandchildren to take over these kinkeeping roles in their turn, and who then reap the benefits by themselves being "kinkept." The contrast between those very old San Franciscans who are family-deprived and those who are family embedded is vivid. Gender differences are apparent, with women more often serving as kinkeepers and caregivers. Old men's family relations are mediated by their wives, old women's by their children. Finally, as Rossi and Rossi (1990) noted for the people they studied at the other end of the country, the closer the kinship connection, the closer the relationship is in old age. Wives and children are more significant than siblings and grandchildren.

References

Aldous, J. (1985). Parent–adult child relations as affected by the grandparent status. In V. L. Bengtson & J. F. Robertson (Eds.), *Grandparenthood: Research and policy perspectives* (pp. 117–132). Beverly Hills, CA: Sage.

Aldous, J. (1987). New views on the family life of the elderly and near-elderly. *Journal of Marriage and the Family, 49,* 227–234.

Bedford, V. (1989). A comparison of thematic apperceptions of sibling affiliation, conflict, and separation at two periods of adulthood. *International Journal of Aging and Human Development, 28,* 53–66.

Bedford, V. (1992). Memories of parental favoritism and the quality of parent–child ties in adulthood. *Journal of Gerontology Social Sciences, 47,* S149–S155.

Bengtson, V. L., & Roberts, R. E. L. (1991). Intergenerational solidarity in aging families: An example of formal theory construction. *Journal of Marriage and the Family, 53,* 856–870.

Bernard, J. (1973). *The future of marriage.* New York: World Press.

Blieszner, R., & Bedford, V. H. (1996). *Aging and the family: Theory and research.* Westport, CT: Praeger.

Glenn, N. D., & McLanahan, S. (1982). Children and marital happiness: A further specification of the relationship. *Journal of Marriage and the Family, 44,* 63–72.

Johnson, C. L. (1993). The prolongation of life and the extension of family relationships: The families of the oldest old. In P. Cowan & D. Field (Eds.), *Family, self, and society: Toward a new agenda for family research.* Hillsdale, NJ: Erlbaum.

Johnson, C. L. (1994). Social and cultural diversity of the oldest-old [Special issue]. *International Journal of Aging and Human Development, 38,* 1–12.

Johnson, C. L., & Catalano, D. (1981). Childless elderly and their family supports. *The Gerontologist, 21,* 610–618.

Johnson, C. L., & Troll, L. (1992). Family functioning in late late life. *Journal of Gerontology Social Sciences, 47,* S66–S72.

Johnson, C. L., & Troll, L. (1994). Constraints and facilitators of friendships in late late life. *The Gerontologist, 34,* 79–87.

Kovar, M. G. (1986, May 1). *Aging in the eighties. Advanced data.* U.S. Department of Health and Human Services (No. 115).

Lamb, H. E., & Lamb, J. E. (1976). The nature and importance of the father–infant relationship. *Family Coordinator, 25,* 379–388.

Litwak, E. (1960). Geographic mobility and extended family cohesion. *American Sociological Review, 25,* 385–394.

Rosenthal, C. J. (1985). Kinkeeping in the familial division of labor. *Journal of Marriage and the Family, 47,* 965–974.

Rossi, A. S., & Rossi, P. H. (1990). *Of human bonding: Parent–child relations across the life course.* New York: Aldine de Gruyter.

Shanas, E. (1979). The family as a social support system in old age. *The Gerontologist, 19,* 169–174.

Shanas, E., Townsend, P., Wedderburn, E., Fries, H., Milhhoj, P. & Stehouver, J. (1968). *Older people in three industrial societies.* New York: Atherton.

Treas, J. (1977). Family support systems for the aged: Some social and demographic considerations. *The Gerontologist, 17,* 486–491.

Troll, L. E. (1983). Grandparents: The family watchdogs. In T. Brubaker (Ed.), *Family relationships in later life* (pp. 63-74). Beverly Hills, CA: Sage.

Troll, L. E. (Ed.). (1986). *Family issues in current gerontology.* New York: Springer.

Troll, L. E. (1994). Family-embedded vs. family-deprived oldest-old: A study of contrasts. *International Journal of Aging and Human Development, 38,* 51–66.

Troll, L. E., & Bengtson, V. L. (1979). Generations in the family. In W. Burr, G. Nye, R. Hill, & I. Reiss (Eds.), *Contemporary theories about the family* (pp. 127–161). New York: Free Press.

Troll, L. E., & Bengtson, V. L. (1992, Summer). The oldest-old in families: An intergenerational perspective. *Generations: Journal of the American Society on Aging,* 39–44.

Troll, L. E., Miller, S. J., & Atchley, R. (1979). *Families of later life.* Belmont, CA: Wadsworth.

Uhlenberg, P., & Cooney, T. N. (1990). Family size and mother–child relations in later life. *The Gerontologist, 3,* 618–625.

■ ■ ■

2

Women and Men "In the Middle": Caregiving and Demographic Changes

Janet Belsky, PhD

When the cohort of men and women who are now in their 50s and 60s were growing up, people could look forward to retirement age as a period of peace from family demands. Children were grown. A "miracle economy" (Krugman, 1994), low divorce rates, and far fewer working women (Furstenberg & Cherlin, 1991; Popenoe, 1988) meant adults were less in need of parents' help after they left home and had children of their own. Because not as many people lived to their 80s and 90s, it was much less common for men and women in late middle age to still have a parent alive (Brody, 1985; Gatz, Bengtson, & Blum, 1990).

Today, these decades have become a time of greater giving to both a more needy older and younger generation. Although this change in the family has been widely publicized, in this chapter I argue that the natural impulse may still be to use the past as a standard for what is happening now. Such a tendency to measure the present by the past produces predictable guilty feelings, adding to the stress women and men feel when they are asked to provide this family help. Counselors need to be alert to these predictable misperceptions, understand why they are likely to arise, and work to educate clients "in the middle" to help them avoid the temptation to misread personal failure into what is really social change.

Caregiving Idea Relating to Aged Parents: "I'm Not Doing Enough"

We know that there has been a dramatic increase in life expectancy during the 20th century. However, clients caring for aged parents may not fully appreciate that over the past 30 years the real revolution has occurred in late-life life expectancy, the number of years people can expect to live after age 65 (Rosenwaike & Dolinsky, 1987; U.S. Senate Special Committee on Aging, 1991). When this cohort of late middle-aged women and men were growing up, people were more likely to live to their sixties and then die, often of a sudden heart attack. Due in part to the fitness movement, in recent decades a marked drop in mortality rates from heart disease (Ettinger, 1994) has occurred, allowing more people to live to their 80s and beyond. When late-life life expectancy increases, people are more vulnerable to chronic illnesses that gradually disable rather than suddenly kill (e.g., Alzheimer's disease, osteoporosis, sensory impairments). The price of recent longevity gains is multiple chronic illnesses and a higher risk of disabilities (Ettinger, 1994; Manton & Suzman, 1992; Verbrugge, 1990)—a frailer older parent generation than before.

The impact on daughters, the primary caregivers for these frail older people, is striking. In polling several hundred women of different ages, researchers (Moen, Robinson, & Fields, 1994) found that while almost two thirds of the women aged 55–64 reported having cared for an aged relative, fewer than half of the women in their parents', age group (people over age 75) had, a 20% rise in the risk of caregiving over one generation. Moreover, because people who live longer are apt to be frailer, caregiving today is likely to be more demanding and go on for a more protracted period than at any time in history.

Daughters who are caregivers may not realize that their mothers may never have actually been caregivers. They are not likely to understand that if their mothers did care for an aged parent, the demands on them were probably less intense. So women compare themselves to their mothers and feel deficient: "My mother never felt ambivalent about caring for an aged mother or father." "She never hired outside help to cope." "She never put her parent in a nursing home." These are false comparisons. The burden of caregiving weighs much heavier today (Brody, 1985; Selig, Tomlinson, & Hickey, 1991).

The idea that "my mother would have handled things differently" not only compounds the overall stress of providing care, it may keep some women (and men) from getting the services they need. Studies show that even when formal sources of help such as home care or day care are available they tend to be used sparingly, not only by spouses but also by caregiving children (U.S. Senate Special Committee on Aging, 1991). One reason is that paid-for services are costly; another reason may be that people are genuinely morally committed to providing care on their own (Selig, Tomlinson, & Hickey, 1991). However, to what degree is this lack of utilization due to misguided conceptions about "the good old days?" To what extent is this need to "do everything myself" based on false ideas about what the previous generation might have done?

This generation's sense of being morally deficient compared with their parents is apt to be heightened by another societal change. When this cohort of women and men in the middle were growing up, families were much more likely to share households. Today, the older generation lives alone. However, this decline in extended family living has nothing do with children caring less. In the past, older people were forced by economic necessity to live with their adult children. In the early 1970s, expanded Social Security and retirement benefits and the institution of Medicare and other entitlement programs meant that older people finally had the financial resources to live on their own (see Shanas, 1979a, 1979b).

Furthermore, the older generation prefers things this way. Surveys show older White European people vigorously reject the idea of intergenerational households (Hamon & Blieszner, 1990; Okraku, 1987). What they want is an arrangement called "intimacy at a distance," living nearby but not together (Shanas, 1979a, 1979b). In other words, although clients (and counselors) may be tempted to use the fact that grandma no longer lives with the family as evidence that children are not as committed as in "the good old days," this too is an erroneous idea.

In fact, studies underline the fact that children are committed to their aged parents (Gatz, Bengtson, & Blum, 1990). For instance, even though family mobility is prevalent, a remarkable amount of elderly parent–adult child contact still takes place in the United States. In 1984, one out of three adults saw an aged parent daily or every other day. Almost two in three reported seeing that person once or twice within the past seven days (Crimmins & Ingegneri, 1990). In a more recent telephone survey (Lawton, Silverstein, &

Bengtson, 1994), two thirds of the people polled reported seeing an elderly mother at least once a week. Most reported that their relationship with their older parent was enduring and close .

Moreover, contrary to the dire stereotypes, families are not dumping their aged parents in nursing homes. For every disabled person in a nursing home, two equally disabled elderly are being cared for by family members, often at great emotional cost (U.S. Senate Special Committee on Aging, 1991). Nursing home placement is something families strenuously work to avoid. Often, it happens as a last resort when a daughter gets ill and cannot provide the care (Brody, 1977). In other words, that other "obvious" sign of children neglecting aged parents, the dramatic rise in the number of long-term care facilities, is also due to demographic, not personal, changes (e.g., a more disabled older population, fewer family members able to provide care).

Caregiving Idea Relating To Adult Children: "I'm Doing Too Much"

Regarding the younger generation, those in the middle are likely to have the opposite feeling: "I am doing more than I should." Again, this emotion is understandable when a person bases his or her criteria of helping on "the way things used be." According to Kuypers and Bengtson (1983), parent–child relationships follow an implicit "norm of waning involvement." As children are growing up they are supposed to need less time and attention from parents. Once they are grown up, they should be fully on their own.

In the past, this norm was easier to follow. Because of changes in the economy and the family, meeting this standard is more difficult for today's young adults. When the cohort of men and women now in their 30s and 40s were growing up during the 1950s and 1960s, it was the older generation who was poor. Now, with the exception of women over 85 living alone, young adults (and their children) are the poorest segment of society, the people who are suffering most from the declining standard of living of the past 20 years (Children's Defense Fund, 1994). Many entry level jobs no longer pay an adequate wage. Working at a minimum wage job for 40 hours a week in 1993, for instance, only put the typical U.S. family of four at 75% of the poverty line (Karger & Stoetz, 1994). Moreover, while in the past young people might have needed their parents' help only when getting established, and then go on to climb the ranks of their permanent jobs, today's workers are more vulnerable, more likely to be laid off and have to change careers or go back to school periodically during their life. This transition from stable employment to what is euphemistically called "boundaryless careers" (Bird, 1994; De Fillippi & Arthur, 1994) means that young adults not only need more help at the beginning, they may have to rely on their more affluent parents at several points throughout their lives.

The rise in one-parent families dramatically increases the chance of dependence. One half of all single mothers and their children live in poverty (Children's Defense Fund, 1994). From the early 1970s to the mid 1980s, the number of mother-headed households doubled from 1 in 10 to more than 1 in 5 (U.S. Bureau of the Census, 1990). This statistic only measures the number of single-parent families at a given point in time. It is estimated that about 60% of all children in America will spend some time in a single-parent family at some point during their growing years (Kamerman & Kahn, 1988).

These changes mean that the norm of waning parental involvement is no longer applicable. It needs to be replaced by a parenting norm that stresses unpredictably waxing and waning help. Waxing parental involvement when an adult child is undergoing life transitions has been best documented in divorce. When a daughter is divorced, the level of mother-to-daughter help rises dramatically. Grandparents step in, helping with finances and child care (Aldous, 1985; Johnson, 1985) . The involvement even extends to the basics of life. An examination of custody cases referred to a Canadian court over a 1-year period found that more than three in four grandchildren had lived in a grandparent's home during this time (Wilks & Melville, 1990).

Once again, when women and men in the middle use their own, more secure life path as their framework, the stress of providing this greater help to children is magnified. People remember what they asked from their parents when they were young adults and feel they are being taken advantage of, that their children are asking too much. Without an understanding of societal changes, they may also blame their sons and daughters for failing at goals that were far easier to accomplish in their own youth. It was easier to be financially independent from parents in an era when higher wage jobs were plentiful and company downsizing was not a fact of life (Bird, 1994). Staying married in the 1950s and 1960s was less difficult, because the social sanctions against divorce were high and the economic stresses on two-parent families less intense. By using their own young adult years as their benchmark, people are not only likely to become angry at their children but also at themselves. In a recent study (Hamon & Cobb, 1993), many parents reported having these self-condemning feelings, at least partly blaming themselves when their children got divorced. Once parents really understand that what is happening has little to do with their own or a child's personal deficiencies, they can get on with the job of providing the support their sons and daughters need.

Conclusion

Counselors who work with clients in this middle generation need to be aware of these misperceptions about caregiving. First, they need to be sensitive to comments by clients comparing the past with the present. Statements such as "My mother would never have done that to her mother," "In our family we always cared for our elderly relatives on our own," "I never asked my mother for help babysitting," or "Why can't my son find a job? After all, he has a college degree" are indications that the client may not fully understand the way society has changed.

Counselors then need to function as "demographic educators," disputing these false analogies by providing information about societal change. The best approach might be to cite statistics such as those used in this article, as well as to draw on the individual's own experience: "Do you recall your grandmother being disabled for months? Did she live to be 90 like your mother has?" "How many of your son's classmates have been able to get high paying jobs?" "How many friends' children have been divorced?" Counselors should help clients understand that they are using the outdated norm of waning involvement and explain why it no longer fits reality.

Clients "in the middle" do need to appreciate their vital role in the family. Today, people in their 50s and 60s are often the bulwark keeping the family afloat. However, because there are no models for how involved one should be, counselors need to emphasize that people in this position have the difficult task of creating their own rules. Counselors can then work to assist clients to construct these personal norms of caregiving unencumbered by an outmoded vision or model of family life.

References

Aldous, J. (1985). Parent–child relations as affected by the grandparent status. In V. L. Bengtson & J. F. Robertson (Eds.), *Grandparenthood* (pp. 117–132). Beverly Hills, CA: Sage.

Bird, A. (1994). Careers as repositories of knowledge: A new perspective on boundaryless careers. *Journal of Organizational Behavior, 15,* 325–344.

Brody, E. (1977). *Long term care of older people.* New York: Human Sciences Press.

Brody, E. (1985). Parent care as a normative family stress. *Gerontologist, 25,* 19–29.

Children's Defense Fund. (1994). *State of America's children (Yearbook, 1994).* Washington, DC: Children's Defense Fund.

Crimmins, E., & Ingegneri, D. C. (1990). Interactions and living arrangements of older parents and their children: Past trends, present determinants, future implications. *Research on Aging, 12,* 3–35.

Defillippi, R., & Arthur, M. B. (1994). The boundaryless career: A competency-based perspective. *Journal of Organizational Behavior, 15,* 307–324.

Ettinger, C. (1994, April). *Healthy aging: How to die with your boots on.* Paper presented at the annual meeting of the Southern Gerontological Society, Charlotte, NC.

Furstenberg, F., & Cherlin, A. (1991). *Divided families.* Cambridge, MA: Harvard University Press.

Gatz, M., Bengtson, V. L., & Blum, M. (1990). Caregiving families. In J. E. Birren & K. W. Schaie (Eds.), *Handbook of the psychology of aging* (3rd ed., pp. 404–426). New York: Academic Press.

Hamon, R. R., & Blieszner, R. (1990). Filial responsibility expectations among adult child–older parent pairs. *Journal of Gerontology, 45,* P110–112.

Hamon, R. R., & Cobb, L. L. (1993). Parents' experience of and adjustment to their children's divorce: Applying family stress theory. *Journal of Divorce and Remarriage, 21,* 73–94.

Johnson, C. L. (1985). Grandparenting options in divorcing families. In V. L. Bengtson & J. F. Robertson (Eds.), *Grandparenthood* (pp. 81–96). Beverly Hills, CA: Sage.

Kamerman, S. D., & Kahn, A. (1988). *Mothers alone: Strategies for a time of change.* Boston, MA: Auburn House.

Karger, H. J., & Stoetz, D. (1994). *American social welfare policy: A pluralistic approach* (2nd ed). White Plains, NY: Longman.

Krugman, P. (1994). *Peddling prosperity: Economic sense and nonsense in the age of diminished expectations.* New York: Norton.

Kuypers, J. H., & Bengtson, V. L. (1983). Toward competence in the older family. In T. H. Brubacker (Ed.), *Family relations in later life* (pp. 211–228). Beverly Hills, CA: Sage.

Lawton, L., Silverstein, M., & Bengtson, V. (1994). Affection, social contact, and geographic distance between adult children and their parents. *Journal of Marriage and the Family, 56,* 57–68.

Manton, K. G., & Suzman, R. (1992). Forecasting health and functioning in aging societies. In M. Ory, R. P. Abeles, & P. D. Lipman (Eds.), *Aging, health, and behavior* (pp. 327–357). Newbury Park, CA: Sage.

Moen, P., Robinson, J., & Fields, V. (1994). Women's work and caregiving roles: A life course approach. *Journal of Gerontology, 49,* S 176–186.

Okraku, I. (1987). Age and attitudes towards multigenerational residence, 1973–1983. *Journal of Gerontology, 42,* 280–287.

Popenoe, D. (1988). *Disturbing the nest.* New York: Aldine de Gruyter.

Rosenwaike, I., & Dolinsky, A. (1987). The changing demographic determinants for the growth of the extreme aged. *Gerontologist, 27,* 275–280.

Selig, S., Tomlinson, T., & Hickey, T. (1991). Ethical dimensions of intergenerational reciprocity: Implications for practice. *Gerontologist, 31,* 624–630.

Shanas, E. (1979a). Social myth as hypothesis: The case of family relations of older people. *Gerontologist,* 19, 3–9.

Shanas, E. (1979b). The family as a social support system in old age. *Gerontologist, 19,* 169–174.

U.S. Bureau of the Census. (1990). *Statistical abstract of the U.S.* Washington, DC: Author.

U.S. Senate Special Committee on Aging. (1991). *Aging America: Trends and projections.* Washington, DC: U.S. Senate Special Committee on Aging and the American Association of Retired Persons.

Verbrugge, L. (1990). The twain meet: Empirical explanations of sex differences in health and mortality. In M. Ory & H. R. Warner (Eds.), *Gender, health and longevity* (pp. 159–199). New York: Springer.

Wilks, C., & Melville, C. (1990). Grandparents in custody and access disputes. *Journal of Divorce, 13,* 1–14.

■ ■ ■

3

Single Older Women and The Family

Dorothy Litwin, PhD

Age is not a good predictor of personality for any individual (Neugarten & Neugarten, 1991). In researching role transitions and goals in old age, Rapkin and Fischer (1992a, 1992b) found that any attempt to establish universal patterns in old age may be an oversimplification. The same may be said for couples and families. The structure of the family is rapidly changing. The variations seen in clinical practice further exemplify the new lifestyles among older women.

- A woman of 79 married a widower a year older than she. This was her third marriage. Independent in many respects, she married a year after she became a widow because she could not tolerate being alone. Although they were sexually involved while courting, she could not countenance living together because she was concerned about her reputation among her friends.

- A 73-year-old woman, divorced by her husband after 48 years of marriage, created a new way of life. She and the widower of a friend see each other regularly on weekends and talk over the phone every day. She finds that she enjoys her own space and time during the week so that she can continue her artistic career and other interests.

- A 62-year-old divorced woman who works and enjoys life is preparing for her married daughters to take over from her the rituals of holidays and celebrations.
- A woman in her early 60s is prevented from having an affair because she is concerned about the possibility of contracting AIDS.

Goldscheider (1990) has shown the manner in which changes in roles in society can bring about changes in behavior. With women entering the work force in greater numbers and able to support themselves, they have become more independent and less apt to tolerate a marginal marriage for economic reasons. When wives work, husbands do not feel as responsible for the economic maintenance of the family and can more easily end a marriage. In addition, women are less likely to marry in order to have children, since unmarried motherhood is now more accepted by society. The couple who is married for a lifetime may be becoming an anachronism

Among the changes in conventional family structure—such as homosexual marriages, single motherhood, and live-in relationships—is the single older woman. The number of single older women is growing. It is important for family therapists to understand how roles and expectations change as women age and to understand the impact this has on their families.

The purpose of this chapter is to examine the role of the older single woman in the family. Changes in society's mores, together with the increasing longevity of women, have affected the role of the older woman in the family. What follows is an attempt to understand her daily life and how she functions.

Demographics

It has been estimated that by the year 2030, one fifth of the population in the United States will be over 65. The overwhelming majority of older people are women, and the likelihood of a woman being single in old age is very high. At chronological age 80, the ratio of women to men is 3:1. A woman can look ahead to approximately one third of her life span without a male mate. While 36% of all men at 80 are married, only 6% of women at 80 are married. The average age of widowhood is 56. Half the women over 65 are widows (McGrath, Keita, Strickland, & Russo, 1990).

Women outlive men an average of 7 years and generally have fewer financial entitlements. After age 65, women spend a greater portion of their lives disabled than do men. These differences result in differing life experiences in old age for women and men. For instance, many married women care for their disabled spouses until their death. Then, after their husbands' death, they live a number of years with personal disability, often while living alone (Chamie, 1991).

Growing numbers of older people are living independently, out of choice, in their own homes. In fact, 50% of women over 65 head their own households. According to a Louis Harris (1990) poll, less than 1% of the elderly who live alone say they would prefer to live with their children, although 75% have children with whom they could live. Of the elderly living alone, 80% are women and two thirds of the elderly living alone are widows (Choi, 1991; Rowland, 1991).

Choi (1991) pointed out that improved economic resources for the elderly (food stamps, social security insurance, cost of living allowances, etc.), changes in the rules and tastes of postindustrial society, and demographic changes in birth rates (i.e., the decrease in the ratio of adult daughters to mothers) are factors that have contributed to the propensity for older people to live alone. However, additional factors involved in the choice are "intergenerational family ties, kinship network, friend interaction, and differing attitude toward privacy, independence and personal freedom" (Choi, 1991, p. 497).

Variations Among Single Women

Increasingly, there are variations in lifestyle among older single women; for instance, some older women chose to be single as a way of life. It is important to note that heterosexual marriage is the stereotype of the older woman and most of the literature is directed along these lines. The widow is the research paradigm and is studied as someone having suffered a loss and having to adjust to a new way of life. How the role of the single woman affects the immediate or extended family is simply not explored, even though this would be an important contribution to family theory. For this reason, what follows is essentially based on clinical experience (Litwin, 1993).

There is a long transitional period between the time a woman becomes single and the time she is in need of caretaking. Not much is known about the impact of this prolonged period of singlehood on the family and the interplay of behavior, expectations, and other needs that surface. Instead, it is as though development stops or stays the same from midlife until the older woman needs caretaking, either from the family or a nursing home. Greenberg (1992) pointed to the number of books written about infants and child development in contrast to the paucity of books about older people. Asking the crucial question about how it is possible to prepare for this stage of life in the community, the family, or individually, Greenberg stated, "It is as though we collude in an unspoken agreement to remain fixed in time, fixed in roles until we go into crises…and then we are unprepared for and shocked at the changes which we are forced to confront" (p. 84).

The present cohort of older women is said to be a pacesetter because there are no role models. Some women seem to be learning from their daughters: The divorce rate among older women is reaching that of the younger generation; older women are becoming involved with significant others as sexual partners; and marriage is not a requirement for many older women.

O'Brien (1991), in studying the life experience of never-married older women, found they did not marry out of choice. Marriage was never a goal for them. Being independent was of greater importance than the security of marriage that our society promises. The study found continuity in satisfaction in life and well-being, indicating stability over the life span as the women grew older.

Some who have been married discover, after being widowed or divorced, that they prefer not to remarry or to be involved with a man, although others find that they cannot bear to be alone. There is a shortage of men: Men marry younger women and men die at younger ages. Many women, like it or not, must become accustomed to being single. Many single older women become involved in social lives with friends and, in fact, seem to have a more active social life than many married older women. Some may choose to develop lesbian relationships at this stage in life.

While loss of spouse and friends through illness and death necessitates role changes, the manner in which the older woman adjusts to these changes depends on her character structure and, in general, how flexible she is in adapting to change. In addition to the loss of an intimate, factors such as retirement, being a victim of ageism, and physical hardship can exacerbate despair concomitant with the role change. The ability to adjust to changing life circumstances reflects prior experiences with stress and loss—not age—even though these events can coincide with growing older.

To be sure, widows and divorcees enter a different world of single women. Widows and divorcees, no longer part of a couple, have to master situations that single women have dealt with all their adult lives. For some a husband is an economic necessity, an escort, a companion, a physical presence; for others, if they are lucky, he is a close, intimate friend. For some, the change from the role of wife to becoming single is the most painful experience in life. For others, the elimination of responsibility for another person and the release from the social obligations and expectations that married life entails are gains that come with being single.

Particularly for the current cohort of older women whose social role was to make the family the center of their lives, being single is especially difficult because they probably did not develop skills to ensure their livelihood and independence. Being part of a couple as a way of life is vital for some. Some stay in bad marriages because of economic reasons, while for others, the social stigma of divorce still exists. For this latter group, change may be difficult because many feel divorce would bring shame and failure to them. Divorce and separation are executed only as a last resort, and then, mostly by men. However, some women can initiate the change, perhaps because circumstances are more propitious or they have more self-confidence, but character, circumstance, social mores, and cultural background have more to do with changes in role than old age. For instance, the extremely dependent older woman is more likely to feel alone and abandoned by the death of her spouse and have greater difficulty in being self-sufficient than another woman who has developed her own interests and has greater inner resources. Some older women relish living alone and not being responsible to or for another human being. That is not to say that even the most well-adjusted single older woman would not have her difficult moments; missing a loving partner may intensify feelings of loss. Whether being alone turns into isolation is characterologically determined.

For some women, divorce or widowhood is certain downward mobility. Within the middle or upper class, or among the more educated, some find new friends and activities while adjusting to their changed status and are absorbed in the ecosystem of their community (Pellman, 1992). Others can continue their lives within the same social circle much as before. Others replace the mate with a man from the same social group, which Lopata (Hess, 1976) called *widow inheritance*. These are solutions that work for some women. For others, being single is preferred as promising and rewarding and perhaps a second chance at a successful way of life. Some may find it necessary to assume this new role contrary to their needs, expectations, or desires. Arriving at successful decisions, whether by default or choice, requires flexibility of character and accommodations made to changing circumstances (Litwin, 1993).

There are endless variations in behavioral patterns that can have an impact on family and friends. Solitude does not necessarily mean isolation. There are some who seem to suffer from being alone. The older woman who has been socialized to live through others and to put her needs second to those of her family is likely to experience loneliness rather than liberation through loss of significant people in her life. This role change to her would, in all likelihood, mean a loss of identity and self-esteem as well as loss of the organizing principle in her life. By contrast, some older women are so independent that they can neither accept nor ask for help; this pretense of being self-sufficient and not needing others can be quite detrimental. Not being involved with others may have always been a way of life for some and isolation may be familiar, if not preferred. Some may appear to be aloof and distant because they are afraid to impose by "asking" and risking rejection. Others may appear remote and detached because intimacy has always been a problem. In addition, there is the "difficult mother" who alienates family members by evoking guilt and anxiety because negative attention is better than none (Litwin, 1993).

Although many single parents live alone, this is not without its effect on the family. Children of single parents may feel responsible for the parent's well-being. Even if there is not a role reversal in which the parent becomes dependent on the child, the child can feel obligated to fill the void for the remaining parent. A promising relationship or marriage for the widowed or divorced parent may be a welcome relief of responsibility for the child. On the other hand, children sometimes interfere with their parent's relationships because of their own conflicts, moral scruples, ageist attitudes, or even pecuniary reasons.

Relationships Of Older Women

It is a misconception that older people become more reclusive and passive with age and that their interpersonal relationships diminish. Research indicates that older people are not more withdrawn: Close emotional relationships are as important as when they were younger. They seek and sustain intimate, interpersonal relationships into their ninth decade, compensating when nuclear family are not alive. Levenson and Carstensen (1993) investigated long-term marriages and found that although there is a reduction in social contacts with age, individuals become increasingly focused on emotionally meaningful relationships. Discussion about children and grandchildren increases as marriages become more companionate.

Armstrong and Goldsteen (1990) concluded that a decline in friendships with chronological age is not every woman's experience but varies considerably with the individual. Levit, Weber, and Guacci (1993) found continuity in social contact: Younger people find friends to be more important; with aging, family becomes more significant. The latter finding was supported by Troll (1994) and Antonucci (1994). Lang and Carstensen (1994) elaborated on this finding and regarded early patterns of close relationships as a foundation for later-life social contact.

Though parents seem to enjoy living near their children and will often move to be geographically closer, the parent–child relationship does not seem to make a difference in the well-being of the older person (Armstrong & Goldsteen, 1990). Having a confidante contributes to survival in old age no matter who that person is. Apparently, it is the quality of the relationship, not the quantity of relationships, that makes the difference. According to a study reported in the *New York Times* (Goleman, 1988), social isolation is as great or a greater risk to mortality than smoking and is as significant as high blood pressure, obesity and cholesterol, or lack of physical exercise.

Looking closely at parent–child families who live together, Speare and Avery (1993) found that most unmarried adult children live with parents because of economics, the need for assistance with the activities of daily living, and ethnicity or race. The authors noted that even though incomes are adequate, Asians as a group have higher coresidence rates than any other racial or ethnic group. This highlights culture as another variable that enters into decisions involving coresidency.

However, as the adult child ages, there is less of a tendency to live with parents, and the female, if she is a single parent, is apt to live independently. As far as the parents go, coresidence declines with the age of the parents, who remain independent until age 85; when the parents need help, there is a decided increase in coresidence.

McCulloch (1990), in investigating which factors are important in the coresidence of intergenerational families, found that reciprocity of services between the generations, whether equal or unequal, failed to make a difference in the well-being of older parents. The researchers posited that factors other than equities or inequities in exchange must be operating that contribute to morale. Hamon and Blieszner (1990) found considerable agreement between older parent–child pairs in expectations of and obligations to one another. The researchers concluded that roles are a dynamic process between the generations.

A different pattern of living arrangements is seen among the widowed and divorced racial minorities. Fewer Black or Hispanic women live alone because they prefer to live with family. Generally, the mother or the grandmother holds the family together; however, there is a great deal of variability among these groups. They do not cherish privacy or independence as much as single White women do, according to Choi (1991). Choi explained further that during racial segregation, social lives took place primarily with the extended family and the same racial group; therefore, people of color continue to find support and comfort within the same social structure.

Developmental Issues Of Older Women

Menopause and the "empty nest" syndrome are reputed to be important turning points in the lives of women; however, as with other events in the lives of women, reactions vary. For some, menopause and children leaving home are liberating events. No longer does one have to be concerned with becoming pregnant and, in fact, sex can be enjoyed more without the fear of pregnancy. Nor does one have to deal with the menstrual cycle and all its complications. Likewise, not having children around and not having the responsibilities of housekeeping and being available as the mother can be very appealing. For some it becomes possible to do all that was put off until the children grew up and were gone. On the other hand, depending on the lifestyle, inner resources, and character structure of the woman involved, either event can be a traumatic turning point.

Many theorists believe, and there is some documentation in the literature, that as couples age, women become more assertive, managerial, and expressive, and men become nurturant, passive, and dependent. A question remains as to whether these role changes come with age or whether changing environmental conditions bring out these latent behaviors. In this regard, Friedman, Tzukerman, Wienberg, and Todd (1992) have concluded that women's power does not increase with age as much as the perception of her power by her mate changes. It is men's status that changes as their roles change and women's supportive roles become more important.

Grambs (1980) believed that sexual behavior undergoes the most pronounced change with aging. Although it is true that there are physiological changes, other contributing factors must be taken into account. For example, drugs prescribed for women, particularly for hypertension, can reduce sexual energy. Though the capacity for arousal and orgasm remains, several factors (e.g., hormones, partner, psychological causes) may affect sexual performance (Leiblum, 1990). In this particular cohort, where many have embraced social stereotypes and believe there is no sex after age 50, a reasonable assumption is that their socialization has made this a self-fulfilling prophecy. Purifoy, Grodsky, and Giambra (1992) found that sexual attitudes and activity decline with age, along with a corresponding increase in negative attitudes. However, they speculated that this effect may have more to do with the paucity of sexual partners than with age. Single life may create methods of adaptation in which "not thinking about it" becomes a solution. However, in my clinical experience, many couples remain active and interested in sex and, in fact, substitute behaviors and devices in order to maintain sexual participation.

Depression And The Older Woman

Depression is common among the elderly. According to McGrath et al. (1990) the incidence among women cannot be determined because methodological difficulties are compounded by medication and physiological conditions. They cited Formanek's 1987 figures of depression among elderly women ranging from less than 2% to 50%.

One of the factors contributing to depression among older women is a loss of control over their lives. Brandstadter and Rothermund (1994) made the point that older people adapt themselves in accordance with how much control they estimate they can have. They adjust their expectations regarding goals, depending on how much mastery they expect to have over their objective. If this is in keeping with the individual's sense of control, it will have a positive effect. Likewise, if the importance to the individual of the particular goal decreases, so will the individual's feeling regarding general control deficits lessen. A sense of control is such an important factor to self-esteem that the individual shifts preferences in order to avoid feeling losses and deficiencies. For example, Roberto and Bartmann (1993) found that those who were able to make their own decisions regarding plans for rehabilitation recovered more completely than those who were dependent on external sources in decision making.

Hollis (1994) found the degree of internal locus of control to be the only important factor related to later-life adjustment. She felt that this may significantly affect individual adaptations to changes in life's circumstances (e.g., retirement, health, losses) and speculated that this may be an important factor in adjustment across the life span.

It should be noted that nursing homes are not geared in this direction; instead, they tend to directly reinforce dependent behavior in elderly residents. In addition, as Rao (1992) pointed out, the power of older persons to run their lives seems to be increasingly vested in impersonal sources as the younger generation is hired in helping positions. Similarly, very few elderly play a role in decision making in voluntary organizations concerned with aging; so even though a feeling of control is important in maintaining self-respect and a sense of autonomy (Kopp & Rozicka, 1993), it is seemingly ignored.

Loss of control can occur when there is a role reversal and adult children take over decision making for their aging parents without consulting them. At best, there is an imbalance in relationships with children, because power resources become limited. Well-meaning family members can help erode the self-esteem of the wife or mother by being overprotective and treating her as though she is incompetent and a dependent child. Ageism, which creates a stereotypic image of the older woman, can get in the way of an objective evaluation of how well the older person is functioning. The power of self-definition is often taken away by well-meaning family members (Roberto & Bartmann, 1993) who are guided by negative attitudes about the elderly rather than by an actual assessment of the functioning of the older woman.

The older woman can try to find ways to maintain her identity in order to avoid compromising herself. In many cases, her "radar" operates to detect nuances in feelings toward her from her children. She may feel as long as she can be of some value to her offspring, she can maintain her autonomy and their respect and approval. If she can supply some kind of service—financial aid, a home, a gathering center, taking care of grandchildren, a source of support for the divorced, widowed, or sick daughter—she will consider herself and be considered useful. As long as she is not dependent on her offspring for particular services and she can find some other means of providing what she needs, she can maintain her autonomy. Because her relationships with her children are so important to her, she will comply or make compromises to avoid risking a conflict, loss, or abandonment. She will sometimes tell her children once a deed is done that she has made a particular decision. Passive resistance is also a useful tool in appearing to comply while actually not doing so. In addition, the aging mother is not above the use of coercion and arousing guilt in her children to maintain contact. Finally, she can resign herself to doing without, so that she need not depend on others to supply her and have power over her.

In an interesting study on rural women in Minnesota, Shenk (1991) found that older women gave as well as received assistance. These women preferred to choose among an informal network of friends and family to help them in various ways, rather than take a chance on the formal system of help where they might lose autonomy and control over decisions. Different people in their social network were chosen for different reasons (e.g., family when sick, strangers for intimate personal care, a particular child or grandchild for emotional support, friends and neighbors for socializing and mutual assistance). The choices made were in accordance with the maintenance of independence and the retention of control over decisions.

Poverty is another factor that contributes to depression in older women. Because women's traditional role has been in the home and not in the commercial workplace, many older women are not vested in pension plans nor are they able to collect much in the way of social security. Minority groups are especially affected. This is particularly so for rural Black women, three fourths of whom live below the poverty line (Kivett, 1993). Many older women are eligible for assistance programs, social security, or Medicaid, but they are often unaware of their eligibility or do not know that such programs exist.

There is a correlation between isolation and poverty. This combination can lead to depression and affect health and behavior, generating a vicious circle. Poverty can be a critical factor in isolation because it limits mobility and access to the outer world. Because of fear, people become confined to apartments in poor neighborhoods where crime rates are generally high. A patient who is a physical therapist and serves Medicaid clients related that it was not unusual for her to be the only visitor some of her patients had seen for days. Another patient who participated in a "help line" to call elderly people was often the only call the recipient had received since the last call. Carlton-LaNey (1992) described how elderly Black farm women whose social lives revolved around church, secret orders, and clubs become isolated because they are no longer able to drive and public transportation is not available. These women then become dependent on others for their social lives and stimulation.

Additional contributing factors to isolation and depression are health and ensuing confinement; divorce; the death of her spouse; children who leave to live lives of their own, sometimes at great geographical distances; retirement from jobs and the loss of those work relationships; and the loss of peers from death, disability, or relocation.

Caregiving And The Older Woman

Caregiving is mostly a woman's responsibility. As the population ages, women are tied to the caregiving role for a very long period of time. Women, in general, are socialized to assume the caregiving role. This assumption is based on rules of obligation to parents, as well as on gender role expectations. Walker (1991) concluded that caregiving is not always freely given and can be a significant source of stress for women and their families.

When caregiving is the primary responsibility of one family member, the caregiver is at greater risk in terms of physical and mental well-being. A national survey estimated that caregivers commit from 5 to 35 hours per week. The *New York Times* (Fein, 1994) had a poignant article describing the roles in which the caregiver finds herself. Not only is she taking care of an older invalid, sometimes for many years, but at the same time, she is growing older herself.

Societal and familial changes can have a significant influence on the caregiver role of women. Two-worker families, common these days as a necessary means of economic support, and divorce limit women's resources as caregivers. In some cases, responsibility to elders is in disagreement with regard for individual desires, independence, and personal fulfillment. The quality of the relationship between the caregiver and the elderly parent, and the close family and the distant family, influences the well-being of the caregiver as well as the older parent (Baker & Hoover, 1993).

Hatch (1991) found interesting differences in caregiving between African American and White women. Hatch found that African Americans often receive help from friends, neighbors, and coworkers—considered part of the extended family network—thus relying less on family members. Hatch suggested that further research be done to determine whether different caregiving hierarchies function for different ethnic or racial groups.

Conclusions

There is very little research on the changing roles of older single women in the family; therefore, I have made an attempt to highlight changes that occur as women age based on clinical experience (Litwin, 1993).

Most older women are single—because they are widowed or divorced, out of preference, or because they have not been able to find a partner. As contemporary society has become more permissive, older women have gained more latitude than ever before and have more choices in how they live their lives. The traditional role is no longer a given. It is important to understand the ways in which single older women affect the family because older, single women are increasing in numbers.

The mother is a pivotal person in the family, generally responsible for the care of children, husband, parents, and friends. The changes that occur once she becomes single have not been explored. Although each woman works out her solution in accordance with her character, personality, and sociocultural influences, growing older is the variable that women have in common. It is important not only to understand how her role changes but also to grasp the reciprocal, dynamic interaction of the older single woman and the family.

To date, the research being done has been basically either personality or trait studies, or a piecemeal approach to a particular variable being investigated. The older woman as an entity is not studied idiographically, or within the context of the family. A useful next step in the understanding of contemporary family dynamics would be to know how the older single woman leads her life.

Future areas of research on single older women should include (a) longitudinal studies of family relationships of single women who choose to be mothers, (b) differences between voluntarily versus involuntarily single older women, (c) power and loss of control issues, (d) sociocultural influences, and (e) the role of gender in aging. Clearly, more research must be undertaken to understand women as they age.

References

Antonucci, T. C. (1994). A life span view of women's social relations. In B. F. Turner & L. E. Troll (Eds.), *Women growing older* (pp. 203-239). Thousand Acres, CA: Sage.

Armstrong, M. J., & Goldsteen, K. S. (1990). Friendship support patterns of older American women. *Journal of Aging Studies, 4*, 391–404.

Baker, G., & Hoover, H. (1993, February). *Research based proportions: Aging and caregiver.* Paper presented at the VI International Interdisciplinary Conference on Women, San Pedro, Costa Rica.

Brandtstadter, J., & Rothermund, K. (1994). Self percepts of control in middle and later adulthood: Buffering losses by rescaling goals. *Psychology and Aging, 9,* 265–273.

Carlton-LaNey, I. (1992). Elderly Black farm women: A population at risk. *Social Work, 37,* 517–523.

Chamie, M. (1991). Aging, disability and gender. *Proceedings of the NGO Committee on Aging Symposium.*

Choi, N. C. (1991). Racial differences in the determinants of living arrangements of widowed and divorced elderly women. *The Gerontologist, 4,* 496–504.

Fein, E. B. (1994, December). Caring at home, and burning out. *The New York Times,* p. B1.

Friedman, A., Tzukerman, Y., Wienberg, H., & Todd, J. (1992). The shift in power with age: Changes in perception of the power of women and men over the life cycle. *Psychology of Women Quarterly, 16,* 513–526.

Goldscheider, F. K. (1990). The aging of the gender revolution. *Research on Aging, 12,* 531–545.

Goleman, D. (1988, August 4). Researchers add sounds of silence to the growing list of health risks. *The New York Times,* p. B7.

Grambs, J. D. (1980). *Women over forty* (Rev. ed.). New York: Springer.

Greenberg, S. (1992, November). *Mutuality in families: A framework for continued growth in late life.* Paper presented at the meeting of the Boston Society for Gerontologic Psychiatry, Inc., Boston, MA.

Hamon, R. R., & Blieszner, R. (1990). Filial responsibility expectations among adult child–older parent pairs. *Journal of Gerontology, 45,* 110–112.

Hatch, L. R. (1991). Informal support patterns of older African-American and White women. *Research on Aging, 13,* 144–170.

Hess, B. B. (Ed.). (1976). *Growing old in America.* New Brunswick, NJ: Transaction Books.

Hollis, L. A. (1994, May). *Women's issues in later adulthood: Psychosocial adjustment, satisfaction, and health.* Poster session presented at the Women's Health Conference, American Psychological Association, Washington, DC.

Kivett, V. (1993). Grandparenting: Racial comparisons of the grandmother role. *Family Relations, 42,* 165–172.

Kopp, R. G., & Rozicka, M. F. (1993). Women's multiple roles and psychological well-being. *Psychological Reports, 72,* 1351–1354.

Lang, F. R., & Carstensen, L. L. (1994). Close emotional relationships in later life: Further support for proactive aging in the social domain. *Psychology & Aging, 9,* 315–324.

Leiblum, S. R. (1990). Sexuality and the midlife woman. *Psychology of Women Quarterly, 14,* 495–508.

Levenson, R., & Carstensen, L. L. (1993). Long term marriage: Age, gender and satisfaction. *Psychology and Aging, 8,* 301–313.

Levit, M., Weber, R., & Guacci, N. (1993). Convoys of social support: An intergenerational analysis. *Psychology and Aging, 8,* 323–326.

Litwin, D. (1993, February). Aging and changing. In D. Litwin (Chair), *Successful aging.* Panel conducted at the VI International Congress on Women, San Pedro, Costa Rica.

Louis Harris and Associates. (1990). *The elderly in five nations: United States, Canada, United Kingdom, West Germany, and Japan.* Survey conducted for the Commonwealth Fund Commission of Elderly People Living Alone, New York.

McCulloch, J. B. (1990). The relationship of intergenerational reciprocity of aid to morale of older parents: Equity and exchange theory comparisons. *Journal of Gerontology, 45,* S450–455.

McGrath, E., Keita, G. P., Strickland, B. R., & Russo, N. F. (1990). *Women and depression.* Washington, DC: American Psychological Association.

Neugarten, B., & Neugarten, D. A. (1991). Policy issues in an aging society (2nd ed.). In M. Storandt & G. VandenBos (Eds.), *The Adult Years: Continuity & Change* (pp. 143–167). Washington, DC: American Psychological Association.

O'Brien, M. (1991). Never married older women: The life experience. *Social Indicators Research, 24,* 301–315.

Pellman, J. (1992). Widowhood in elderly women: Exploring its relationship to community integration, hassles, stress, social support, and social support seeking. *International Journal of Aging and Human Development, 35,* 253–264.

Purifoy, F. E., Grodsky, A., & Giambra, L. M. (1992). The relationship of sexual daydreaming to sexual activity, sexual drive, and sexual attitudes for women across the life-span. *Archives of Sexual Behavior, 21,* 369–385.

Rao, M. (1992). Aging policies and programs: New century—new hopes—new challenges. *Journal of the International Federation on Aging, 19,* 1–10.

Rapkin, B. D., & Fischer, K. (1992a). Framing the construct of life satisfaction in terms of older adults' personal goals. *Psychology and Aging, 7,* 138–149.

Rapkin, B. D., & Fischer, K. (1992b). Personal goals of older adults: Issues in assessment and prediction. *Psychology and Aging, 7,* 127–137.

Roberto, K. A., & Bartmann, J. (1993). Factors related to older women's recovery from hip fractures: Physical ability, locus of control, and social support. *Health Care for Women International, 14,* 457–468.

Rowland, D. (1991). A five nation perspective on the elderly. *Health Affairs, 11,* 205–215.

Shenk, D. (1991). Older rural women as recipients and providers of social support. *Journal of Aging Studies, 5,* 347–358.

Speare, A., Jr., & Avery, R. (1993). Who helps whom in older parent–child families. *Journal of Gerontology, 48,* S64–S73.

Troll, L. E. (1994). Family connectedness of old women: Attachments in later life. In B. F. Turner & L. E. Troll (Eds.), *Women growing older* (pp. 141–169). Thousand Oaks, CA: Sage.

Walker, A. (1991). The relationship between the family and the state in the care of older people. *Canadian Journal of Aging, 10,* 94–112.

■ ■ ■

4

Later-Life Parenthood

A. Rodney Nurse, PhD

A couple of years ago at the beginning of my son's freshman year in high school, I attended an open house for parents of new students. As part of this process, I sat through teacher presentations in each of his classrooms. While listening with one ear to his algebra teacher, I entertained myself by counting the number of fathers who were, like me, gray and in some stage of significant balding. I was surprised and reassured to find myself in the majority of men. This experience started me thinking about the whole business of having children later in life. I began paying attention to my personal experience, listening to my older clients with children still growing up, and keeping my ears and eyes open for broader bases of knowledge with which to inform my work with these older parents.

From 1946 to 1964 births increased by 55% over the previous 19-year period (Dychtwald & Flower, 1989). In 1995, this 19-year cohort averaged 40 years of age. This statistic, along with the recent tendency among the more economically advantaged to delay the age of marriage and having children, provides the basis for anticipating a bulge of older parents in clinicians' offices.

This chapter reflects the involvement and motivation stemming from that original (shining) moment in my son's classroom. As the population ages, the need increases for clinicians to have ways to think about and work with families headed by older parents. This chapter presents a number of parenting issues for consideration by therapists. Although the focus is on the middle to upper-middle-class client population, reference is made to across-the-board demographic data and to longitudinal studies involving representative samples of the U. S. population.

When a couple has children later, the initial process of becoming a family after being a couple, "the great divide" as the Cowans (1992) called it, may take on a different cast. As noted by the Cowans and by Wallerstein (1995), this is a time of great change, crisis, and often marital difficulty. During this transition between life as a couple and life as a triangle, if the couple is rigid, too "set in their ways," they may attempt to maintain their former patterns. This may involve including the child primarily when it is convenient for them, to the detriment of the child. On the other hand, if they have flexible coping styles so that they bend, adapt, and become a new configuration—a true triangle—this augers well for the child's development and their own as well. It may be that some younger parents have less defined dyadic patterns before having a child, making the shift to the family threesome easier.

Family Connections

Older parents are likely to be less overtly dependent on their own parents. Many, especially women, are likely to be caretakers for their own parents (Clausen, 1993). With truly elderly or deceased grandparents, the parents will have less extended family support. Thus "the family" is somewhat more likely to focus on the immediate two-generational structure and less likely to be actively augmented by the third, or grandparent, generation. Older parents who are able to reinforce each other positively and behave self-reliantly have the potential for developing a family environment of achievement and personal responsibility, serving as positive role models for their children. In contrast, younger parents who may have more dependent patterns will have significant trouble as they lean on their children. Older parents have matured; they are likely to be sturdier parents. (Of course, age does not automatically result in maturity.)

A child with older parents may miss being directly connected to a wise and loving grandparent. A child may miss having a grandparent who might compensate for a parent's shortcomings, or who might simply have other assets not present in either parent. On the other hand, a few grandparents are just as mean or self-absorbed as are a few parents, so for some children not having grandparents could be an advantage. Overall, though, children of older age parents will miss the personal experience and historical dimension of the three-generation family.

Time and Money

Some older parents, at least entrepreneurs and professionals, may have an increasingly realistic choice of how and when they commit time. Parents can be more readily available when needed by the child—whether the child is ill, needs a parent to attend the school play, or is having difficulty in school. This flexibility is especially helpful when a child is young. Availability is a prime advantage for a child whose parents have more choice with their scheduling. Some older parents have sufficient autonomy to be able to divide between themselves the various family role functions of a middle-class parent, such as chauffeur, assistant physician, homework consultant, coach, and just good listener, in a way that would not have been easily possible at an earlier career stage.

Because the parents are farther along in their individual life cycles, both may be established in full-time work activity requiring the need for daycare and babysitters for their children or, if they have the resources, nannies or au pairs. This may result in a more buffered environment for the parents and a wider number of people with whom the children will need to relate. Research has consistently indicated that children develop multiple attachments to caregivers who can help them cope with separation anxiety and stress (Ainsworth, 1979; Bray, 1991; Sroufe & Ward, 1984). Children do not need to be reliant on only two caretaking parents.

Of course other circumstances are quite possible. One single parent, through astute financial dealings, was able to retire at 40 and adopt children into her evolving single-parent family.

There is a general trend for people to become more financially secure as they age and develop continued employment success, whether at the blue- or white-collar level. Older parents may have more discretionary income available with which to expand their children's learning opportunities than younger parents might have. In some families, however, increased income or at least a more stable financial base can also give the child an unrealistic idea about the availability of money as he or she moves through adolescence.

One older client, a top executive with a Fortune 500 corporation, lost his job in a restructuring. Instead of concern, he was actually relieved that he and his family would need to relocate to a different part of the country. He knew he would have to cut back on his lifestyle. He believed that this move would demonstrate to his children the reality of money and the real world. He anticipated, too, that he would gain in stature as the prime breadwinner in the family rather than being taken for granted. On subsequent communication from him, he reported that he found the financial struggle difficult but felt his family appreciated his efforts more than when he had seemingly more worldly status and success.

Developmental Issues

Midlife crisis is an issue often raised in connection with older parents (Levinson, 1978; Osherson, 1986). The best available information, however, taken from a 60-year longitudinal study of a large and reasonably representative sample, did not identify midlife as a time of crisis any more than any other time of life (Clausen, 1993). The specter of older parents during this middle span of life being so upset, self-involved, or worried that they may neglect their children is an unwarranted generalization.

Evidence for the "empty nest" syndrome also seems to exist primarily among selected clinical problem samples, not the general population. The Berkeley Longitudinal Studies (Clausen, 1993) found no "empty nest" syndrome. Instead, their subjects tended to report feelings of freedom and relief when their children left home. Sometimes, however, an older couple, having achieved in many areas and having come to grips with not achieving in other areas may, if their relationship is seriously flawed, focus on their child as the meaning for living. The adolescent or young adult may stay with the parents, in part unconsciously, in order to give them a reason for living. While overtly seeming to try to emancipate, the offspring may get into some sort of trouble that inhibits development, such as poor college grades or involvement with drugs. The latter especially provides an anesthetic preventing painful soul-searching followed by growth. In this situation the parents can keep being active parents and do not have to come to grips with their own relationship and aging.

A client in his early twenties with a manic-depressive mother of 60 and a retired father in his 70s was such a case. His mother kept threatening suicide at those times when the young man showed signs of going out with friends and behaving more independently. Her psychiatrist treated her as a manic-depressive, but not as the member of a family. The father found good reason to continue to be involved, helping his son whenever it was called for by the son's problem behavior. At times the father and son focused energy on mother when her depressive episodes occurred, but otherwise she tended to be ignored, seeming to be "well." Only after many sessions of individual therapy did the young man develop insight into his behavior as a way of involving his parents. He feared mightily that his mother would kill herself should he become more independent. While the young man improved with individual therapy and the mother was managed on medication, the family and the psychiatrist, reinforced by managed care restrictions, inadvertently colluded to prevent a family therapeutic intervention.

Another variant on the outcome of excessive child focus by older parents is an inflated sense of self-importance on the part of the child. This may result naturally from an excessive emotional investment on the part of older parents, or it may be the transmission of specific messages to achieve some of the parents' unfulfilled dreams. The child may develop narcissistic behaviors covering over feelings of inferiority. Older parents may be somewhat more vulnerable to falling into this overindulging, flawed parenting pattern.

Parental Characteristics

Whatever age the parents, those who are judged to be good parents possess consistent characteristics that appear repetitively in the literature (Schutz, Dixon, Lindenberger, & Ruther, 1989). These reported characteristics are as follows:

1. A positive emotional attachment communicated to the child.
2. Recognizing of the child as being separate, promoting that autonomy, and placing the child's needs before the parent's.
3. Perceiving the child and his or her uniqueness with accuracy.
4. Parental positive self-esteem and realistic self-confidence.
5. Knowledge of general developmental needs of the child.
6. Flexible responding to the child's behavior.
7. Two-way, open communication, with clarity and respect.
8. Consistent enforcement of appropriate rules and standards.

Assuming positive adult development, these characteristics are more likely to be found in older parents than at least very young ones. On the other hand, if development has been impeded, three major risks for deficient parenting can be present: alcohol and drug addiction, abusive behavior, and severe emotional disturbance.

Sometimes life circumstances and career choices may affect later-life parenting. For example, a professional man in his mid-50s and his 50-year-old wife, who were developing a small business, came to therapy with a marital conflict. He appeared rigid, compulsive, and distant in style, and she tended to be histrionic and labile. Both were furious about not getting what they wanted from each other. She laid the blame on his absorption in his career. In a fit of anger he had hit her. Their teenage daughter was a battleground for the differences between them. He insisted the daughter must achieve academically in order to get into a "good university." She focused on wanting her daughter to gain social skills. For her, the daughter was a rival for the father's attention, even though it was negative attention. At times, though, mother would collude with her daughter against father. The daughter, by keeping herself in the middle of the triangle maintained a balance in the family, headed off the possibility of divorce, and kept the family together.

Conclusion

Demographic information indicating a very significant increase in the number of middle-aged people, coupled with the trend (in at least middle- and upper-class income groups) to marry and have children later, points to the likelihood that therapists and counselors will increasingly see families headed by older parents. Hopefully, the wisdom gained from living longer will mean that more older parents will possess the attitudes and characteristics that research has shown to be identified with "good enough" parents.

There is no need to anticipate a crisis at the parent's midlife. A crisis is no more expected than at any other time in life, according to longitudinal research. And as for the "empty nest" syndrome, longitudinal research suggests it too is nonexistent. In its place, one more likely finds expressions of relief.

Research and clinical observation indicate that for older parents, as with younger, the transition from being a couple to a threesome is a major one. At the same time, there is less intergenerational family support for older parents, since grandparents of the growing child are themselves either older and needing care themselves or deceased. However, research indicates that multiple attachments beyond the traditional nuclear family are good for children. Even though grandparents may not be available, multiple positive attachments, such as with day-care workers, coaches, and babysitters, can greatly enrich a child's experience. Most important, the focus of consulting with families headed by older parents needs to be on the family's uniqueness, even while paying attention to the issues of family connections, aspects of time and money, developmental dimensions, and parental characteristics.

References

Ainsworth, M (1979). Infant–mother attachment. *American Psychologist, 34*, 932–937.

Bray, J. (1991). Psychosocial factors affecting custody and visitation arrangements. *Behavioral Sciences and the Law, 9*, 419–437.

Clausen, J. (1993). *American lives.* New York: Free Press.

Cowan, C. P., & Cowan, P. A. (1992). *When partners become parents.* New York: Basic Books.

Dychtwald, D., & Flower, J. (1989). *Age wave.* Los Angeles: Jeremy P. Tarcher.

Levinson, D. (1978). *The seasons of a man's life.* New York: Knopf.

Osherson, S. (1986). *Finding our fathers.* New York: Free Press.

Schutz, B., Dixon, E., Lindenberger, J., & Ruther, N. (1989). *Solomon's sword.* San Francisco: Jossey-Bass.

Sroufe, L. A., & Ward, M. J. (1984). The importance of early care. In D. Quarm, K. Borman, & S. Gideonse (Eds.), *Women in the workplace: The effects on families* (pp. 35–60). Norwood, NJ: Ablex.

Wallerstein, J. (1995, February). *Remarks on divorce research.* Association of Family and Conciliation Courts, California Chapter Annual Meeting, Sonoma, CA.

■ ■ ■

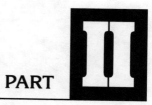

AGING AND FAMILIES: CONFLICTS AND CRISES

5

Reflections of a Therapist and Grandparent: Professional and Personal

Helen M. Strauss, PhD

Grandparenting, along with all other issues of importance to elders, has come into focus nationally as the overall health of elders has improved. As they live longer, elders are being asked increasingly to actively participate in the massive changes that have taken place in our society, changes that make surrogate parenting a given in the lives of many children, and more active grandparenting an unexpected reality for many.

When conditions of work, single parenthood, or the unavailability of either parent prevail, grandparents are more and more frequently pressed to fill the breach. This can be a boon to those whose health and attitudes toward themselves and family combine to make caregiving a desirable option. To others, perhaps less fortunate in health or less equipped in attitude to be caregivers, it is more likely felt to be a burden.

A colleague's two-pronged request motivated me to write this chapter. "Write about grandparent issues in therapy, and their implications for treatment, be it in family or individual therapy," she said, "and write about yourself too, as an older therapist and about how your age affects your work." Since the professional and personal selves are inseparable to me, I will combine them in what follows.

An awesome spectrum invites endless rumination, but I will counter the stereotypic view of the garrulous elderly woman by focusing on a few issues that are most salient to me. On the personal side, how I am seen, as reflected in the sources and nature of the referrals that I receive, is understandably at the forefront. Am I viewed as particularly appropriate to treating other elderly folks, to treating couples, or families? Or, perhaps, there is no discernable pattern of referrals related to being elderly.

A second, and far more important, concern is the growing importance of the elderly as surrogate parents, given the fundamental and far-reaching changes in family life cutting across all socioeconomic and class groups in today's Western societies. The elderly as role models, grandparents, and so forth is a related, though still separate, area of interest and importance. The dramatic and consistent increase in the population's longevity suggests fascinating questions that cry out to be researched.

Finally, the meaning of these unprecedented developments in the modern world to the psychological growth potential of elderly persons can be mind-boggling.

The "Elder" Self as Therapist

Logic would have it that a goodly proportion of an older therapist's referrals and clients in a private practice would be elderly. However, fewer than one third of the clients in my practice are over 65. When an older individual is referred, it is usually at the behest of a son or daughter. Therapy is often doomed from the start, since the patient's own motivation is questionable at best and zero at worst.

A recent such referral lasted three sessions. Belle came, not wishing to be seen as negativistic, and proved willing to describe her listlessness and lack of interest in her current life as an inconsolable widow. Her eyes lit up, however, as she recounted her past, unabashedly alluding to her leadership ability, her business acumen, and her attractiveness as a "man's woman." Currently, her days were occupied with self-serving activities that yielded diminishing returns of interest, let alone joy.

What a waste, I thought. Total narcissistic involvement, and not a thing wrong with her. Her husband's death had left her feeling so deprived and narcissistically injured that no psychic energy was left over to spark generativity. Toward the end of the third session she looked me in the eye, saying, "You can't help me, can you?" My response was that, as Belle knew, help could come only from within herself. We agreed that she was fully aware that she had abundant inner resources, as well as opportunities offered by her environment, for activities that would help dissipate her self-absorption.

To myself I said, "Chalk up another elder who was urged to seek therapy with me by a well-meaning 'other,' simply because I, too, am an 'elder.'" Most such referrals, in my experience, never show up at all or, if they do, leave as soon as they find that problem solving is something they can do just as well for themselves. Why pay a therapist, especially one who seems to constantly throw the ball back into their court?

A very different climate pervaded the treatment of Tanya, a Ukrainian woman of my own age. She came willingly, at her daughter's suggestion. Depression accompanied by insomnia, anxiety attacks, and nightmares were the symptoms that emerged when she moved into her daughter's home in New Jersey, leaving her long-time home base. The deaths of her husband and mother almost simultaneously meant not only their loss but also the loss of her home and professional identity as a musician and teacher.

Several sessions with her "new" family—daughter, son-in-law, and two latency-aged grandsons—gave convincing evidence of the genuinely loving, welcoming spirit pervading her inclusion in the family's life, which she had described. The characterization of close family relationships, transcending mere duty-bound obligation to elders in Eastern European families, was movingly enacted in the family sessions (McGoldrick, Pearce, & Giordano, 1982). Tanya corroborated the same in our individual work.

She sensed my interest in the drama of her life in war-torn Europe and appeared one day with her journal, asking for help in translating it into English so that her grandchildren would be able to read it.

As my vacation time approached after many months of therapy, Tanya expressed her eagerness for my return as soon as possible to complete the translation and editing of her journal. Gone was her need for a therapist, replaced with an urgent wish for an empathic collaborator. Was this therapy? Emphatically yes. The art of listening can take many forms. The fact that my life span and personal interests had covered the same period as hers had made it possible for her to work through her issues of loss and to adapt positively to her new life.

The conclusion to be drawn from these two contrasting cases is that elderly patients react idiosyncratically, reflecting the particular interpersonal dynamics generated in the therapeutic relationship.

The "Elder" Self as Grandparent

The traditional middle-class stereotype—of the grandparent as more benign and indulgent than the parents—cannot be maintained when grandparents become the primary caregivers, even if caregiving is only on a part-time basis. When parents are not present to perform the limit setting, the disciplining, the community- and school-relating jobs, many grandparents are pressured to take over. In the study by Erikson, Erikson, and Kivnick (1986), an interview with one grandmother demonstrated the most positive attitude—on the continuum from unequivocal rejection to joyous acceptance—of the surrogate parenting role:

> She came to appreciate the chance to perform, again, the activities she had found so gratifying as a mother, and the unique opportunity to become as close to her grandson as she is now. She recalls, 'I was his Mom. He called me Mom. I took him to nursery school with a bunch of kids. I PTA-d all over again—in my late sixties, this was.' (p. 94)

Opportunities for tensions, dysfunctions, and frustrations in situations less benign than this are obvious. When therapy is sought, the patient is more often the grandchild than the parenting grandparent, for it is the child who often responds by acting out. Anger, generated by the loss or absence of the parent, can be manifested in myriad ways. Acting out is the least toxic, perhaps, as the depression that many children experience often goes unnoted. Research and case material are sparse on this issue but can be inferred from the fairly numerous studies on cultural and ethnic issues in family therapy.

When grandparents become parents, we must assess the relative strength of countervailing forces: the traditional attitudes of indulgence and the deeper layers of pride in children who will continue the families' bloodlines, versus the negative feelings of being imposed on at a time of life that had been anticipated as leisurely. The latter situation is often exacerbated by the realistic factors of aging minds and bodies, which make the parenting of children a taxing job.

To parent an infant is certainly a strenuous job; caring for toddlers is even more so. Adding the psychological stressors of the child's necessary, healthy, assertive, and often oppositional behaviors which enable age-appropriate separation-individuation can be overwhelming. The stereotypically benign relationship existing between individuals separated by two generations can become less than positive. Widely differing value systems come into play and may tend to be played out in mutually rejecting, negatively judgmental attitudes.

The grandparent generation assumes focal importance when cultural–ethnic factors are involved in therapy, be it individual or family. In my practice, interfaith and interethnic marriages, which have been on the increase nationally, are often the core issues in this category. A considerable literature documents diverse approaches (Grambs, 1989; Haley, 1987; Ingersoll-Dayton, Arndt, & Stevens, 1988; McGoldrick et al., 1982; Minuchin, 1981). The grandparent, as the major carrier of tradition, often regulates by virtue of that powerful cultural vector innumerable aspects of family atmosphere and behavior. When an elder misuses the tyranny of tradition as a power weapon, the pain in all three generations involved can be immeasurable.

Grandparents as Role Models

Looking back at the grandmother role model in my own life, I still sense my pride in the legendary figure described to me by my mother of her own mother who had died long before I was born. A 19th-century European woman, she had been a peace activist, a professional writer, a musician, and an artist. She was also a woman who had borne seven children and suffered four additional pregnancies that ended in stillbirths. She was certainly a feminist before the term was coined and, just as certainly, a determining influence on the development of my mother and of me.

The fact that she has exerted a strong influence on my attitudes as a woman via my mother and, into the fourth generation, on those of my daughter is evidence of the vital importance of generational patterns in the formation of character and personality. How these constants are played out in the kaleidoscopic mosaic of social change is never-endingly fascinating and offers fertile fields for research.

Clinical–Developmental Issues for a Grandparent-Therapist

Do patients' transference manifestations change as the therapist ages? Several patients come to mind, all of whom held grandmothers as major benign figures in their lives.

Robert, a young man of 24, still revelled in the memory of a grandmother who had died when he was two and a half. She had praised him for his exploits of physical derring-do and for bringing her orange juice. To me he was able to recount his derring-do in business dealings with braggadocio when he triumphed and with equally grandiose grief when he failed. He was able to acknowledge his drug and alcohol addictions and his failures in sexual exploits. The transference to me as a benign gray-haired grandmother figure was indelibly clear. He developed a tenderly trusting feeling toward me early in therapy, enabling him to confront the characterological flaws that repeatedly sabotaged his grandiose success schemes.

Colleen, a 30-year-old married mother of two young children, formed an intense attachment to me so quickly after beginning therapy that a transferential explanation was obvious. And there, in clear silhouette, was grandmother. She was remembered as the only unconditionally loving parental figure in her life. Colleen had been sexually and emotionally abused by an older brother from childhood into adolescence. She was unprotected by her parents who idolized the brother and turned a deaf ear to her complaints. Comfort came only from the grandmother, whose benign role in Colleen's life opened the door to therapy on the wave of a powerful positive grandmother transference.

Eric, 7 years old, mourned his grandmother who had recently died. His parents, though loving, had little time for him, as they both worked. Eric was fobbed off on housekeepers who likewise had little time for him. His teacher recommended therapy, because Eric was acting out inappropriately. From the very first session, Eric loved coming to see me. Early in treatment he asked my age and, upon being told it, said, "You should be dead." Being able to discuss with Eric the fact that my being as old as his grandmother had been did not mean that I, too, had to die helped him to deal with his grief and anger.

Several family sessions were conducted, yielding ample insight into the dynamics of parents stressed almost beyond tolerance by the need to sustain a "yuppie" lifestyle in an upper-middle-class community, with little energy or motivation to attend to a 7-year-old, let alone understand his needs for love and attention. He was truly a neglected child whose parents soon found it too onerous to bring him to therapy, since treatment was not covered by their insurance.

In their attitudes toward Eric, as well as toward their own place in the new community, they exemplified what McGoldrick calls "transitional conflict" (McGoldrick et al., 1982, p. 556). Assimilation and success in competing with the community was accompanied by extreme stresses of overwork, loss of warmth in relating to each other, and depression that indicated unworked-through feelings of loss. Eric was the sad victim of these multifaceted stressors.

We move now from the positive transference to the negative. As immortalized by the Wicked Witch of the West in *The Wizard of Oz* and all other gray-haired hags who ride broomsticks on Halloween, grandmothers can be fearsome creatures.

Linda, who suffered from chubbiness in childhood, was unfortunate to have been the only daughter of a mother who was obsessed with weight consciousness, superintending every bite her daughter ate. Her grandmother, too, was so anxiety-ridden about food intake that when she brought cookies to her grandchildren, she would permit Linda only a half a cookie. Linda, now a successful attorney, married and the mother of two, still cringed at the thought of mother and grandmother eyeing her disapprovingly, should she gain an ounce. She herself was the prisoner of the same obsession, superintending her own and her children's eating as intently as she was taught to do. The ambivalence, rage, and impotence she still experienced from these early relationships manifested themselves in the grandmother–mother transference reactions to me: She alternated postures of listening slavishly to my every word and of tuning me out completely. Finally, as if exhausted by 4 years of ricocheting between positive and negative feelings, she quit.

Research and Follow-Up

Research and treatment can often, and at times ideally, go hand-in-hand. The work of Kornhaber and Woodward (1981), Erikson, Erikson, and Kivnick (1986), and Kivnick (1982) are excellent examples of this approach.

Practitioners supply their hands-on knowledge of dynamic issues between grandparents, children, and grandchildren. Social psychologists design questionnaires that access attitudes, the nature of interactions, communication patterns, intrafamilial power lines, and ethnic and class characteristics and differences. The dynamic, clinical, and developmental issues described above could designate the major foci of questionnaires. Ideally, longitudinal follow-up would yield data regarding the facts and perceptions of the grandparenting role, reflecting ongoing changes in society.

One example of societal change, barely researched and most worthy of note in the Western world today, is the grandparent of an adopted child. Children are being sought for adoption increasingly, not only by heterosexual married couples but also by single adults and homosexual and lesbian couples as well. What are the feelings and relationships of family members in these circumstances? Blum (1983) dealt solely with the traditional picture of the middle-class Caucasian couple adopting a Caucasian child. However, his sensitive analysis of the multifaceted feelings that can emerge in the three generations involved can be extrapolated validly to any of the nontraditional conditions prevalent today.

> Considering the transmission of communications about adoption, one has to take three generations into account. …If the grandparent does not regard the adopted child as a true grandchild, this will have an impact upon parent and child. Grandparent and parent may regard the child both as an exception and as an 'outsider' and unconsciously condemn and reject the child as born in sin and out-of-wedlock, viewing the child as the product of the "wild seed" of a delinquent or prostitute mother. The adopted child, assuming his abandonment by his natural parents, may feel that he is the bad seed of "bad parents," but this fantasy may also be shared and mediated in unconscious communications from parents and grandparents. (p. 147)

Clearly, the probability of negative interactions and communications, stemming from the dynamics that Blum delineates, are likely to be intensified in nontraditional adoptive arrangements. These are dynamics that must affect our practice and affect our own lives as grandparents. They require the utmost in self-scrutiny, especially because we are elderly and have been reared, more likely than not, in a more rigid system of values than the norms governing our children's values today.

Hargrave and Anderson (1992) discussed future issues that research and technique in family therapy will, of necessity, be forced to confront. Their conclusion echoes mine:

> As we near the end of the 20th century, the contrast between the elderly's position in 1900 and the elderly's position in 1992 is marked. The many changes that have occurred over the last 90 years now present family therapists with new challenges as we move toward the 21st century. (p. 190)

Grandparents and "The Fourth Individuation"

Kivnick (1982) summed up the findings of her wide-ranging interview study as follows:

The life-cycle importance of grandparenthood suggests that meaningful grandparent-grandchild contact is likely to be of value to family members in all generations. In addition to its consequences during childhood, the absence of a meaningful childhood relationship with a grandparent may well limit the richness of the relationships a given individual will have with grandchildren, two generations into the future. (p. 150)

Examining my own motivations as a grandparent, I experience needs to be nurturing, to have that second chance to improve on the parenting that helped shape my own children's development. Conversely, I hold back, hesitating to intrude on parent–child relationships by introducing unaccustomed indulgences or limits. Even as I write these words, however, I hear myself asking, "Am I, with this hands-off stance, contributing to that societal attitude that devalues the elderly, doesn't really hear them when they speak?" Wainrib (1992) cited several authors whose research has shown this devaluation to be a significantly pervasive pattern. Better, I say to myself, to leave my grandchildren with the image of a competent, responsible individual who acts out of her own personhood than to be remembered as a wimpish nonentity.

My grandchildren will hopefully one day occupy the five-generational vantage point that I now enjoy: memories of parents and grandparents, alongside the here-and-now relationships with their own children and grandchildren—the unending chain along which traditions, culture, and genes are transmitted.

What will be the most effective theoretical models with which to intervene when family therapy is the modality of choice in dealing with the ever-increasing numbers of aging families? New constellations of the family itself will require creative revisions of current methodologies. Griffin (1993) noted in his compendium,

Multigenerational family therapy theorists are similar to object relations theorists in their emphasis on the individual's intrapsychic evolution. Primary differences are the additional emphasis on the multigenerational transmission of pathology and on individuation from the family of origin. (p. 76)

Margaret Mahler (1974) described how the breaking of the symbiotic tie between mother and infant is as inevitable as biological birth. That same sense of irreversible change, for child and parent, is evident during the third individuation. Normal, sexually mature children will inevitably leave their parents and reproduce, thrusting the parents into a new relationship with another child who is a further genetic extension of themselves. The result of this new relationship, which can have such a powerful enriching effect on the middle-

and late-life development of the new grandparents, is the fourth individuation.

Colarusso's paper (1990) on "the third individuation" has provided me with an excellent conclusion to the foregoing reflections:

Intimations of the Fourth Individuation

When their child becomes a parent, new grandparents must redefine their standing among the generations, alter their internal representations of their 'child,' and develop new object ties to the grandchild. Because they are struggling with the middle- and late-life developmental tasks of dealing with retirement, illness, deaths of friends or spouse, and other experiences attending normal aging, new grandparents are developmentally primed to turn their attention toward children and grandchildren, objects who represent their (genetic) future, a future that will endure even after death, the final separation. (p. 193)

As therapists of the grandparent generation, whatever our theoretical persuasion, we share a common goal: to enhance the quality of life for these clients as they approach life's final chapters. I will end on a personal note. The notion of the fourth individuation is a fine one for me, as it assumes that positive change is possible at a stage of life that has stereotypically been seen as rigid and narcissistically depressed. Increasingly, we experience in our work grandparents who are serving as surrogates for parents when divorce, addictions, or other disruptive forces compel them to become the virtual parents.

As therapists, it is essential to view our elderly clients, in family or individual work, as having the capacity to adapt to the rapid, radical changes that continue to redefine family life.

References

Blum, H. P. (1983). Adoptive parents' generative conflict and generational continuity. In A. J. Solnit, R. S. Eissler, & P. B. Neubauer (Eds.), *The psychoanalytic study of the child* (Vol. 38, pp. 141–164). New Haven, CT: Yale University Press.

Colarusso, C. A. (1990). The third individuation: The effect of biological parenthood on separation-individuation processes in adulthood. In A. J. Solnit, P. B. Neubauer, S. Abrams, & A. S. Dowling (Eds..), *The psychoanalytic study of the child* (Vol. 45, pp. 179–194). New Haven, CT: Yale University Press.

Erikson, E., Erikson, J., & Kivnick, H. (1986). *Vital involvement in old age.* New York: Norton.

Grambs, J. D. (1989). *Women over forty.* New York: Springer.

Griffin, W. (1993). *Family therapy: Fundamentals of theory and practice.* New York: Brunner/Mazel.

Haley, J. (1987). *Problem-solving therapy: New strategies for effective family therapy.* New York: Jossey-Bass.

Hargrave, T. D., & Anderson, W. T. (1992). *Finishing well: Aging and reparation in the intergenerational family.* New York: Brunner/Mazel.

Ingersoll-Dayton, B., Arndt, B., & Stevens, D. (1988). Involving grandparents in family therapy. *Journal of Contemporary Social Work, 69*(5), 280–288.

Kivnick, H. (1982). *The meaning of grandparenthood.* Ann Arbor: University of Michigan Research Press.

Kornhaber, A., & Woodward, K. L. (1981). *Grandparents/grandchildren: The vital connection.* Garden City, NY: Doubleday.

Mahler, M. (1974). Symbiosis and individuation: The psychological birth of the human infant. In R. S. Eissler, A. Freud, M. Kris, & A. J. Solnit (Eds.), *The psychoanalytic study of the child* (Vol. 29, pp. 89–106). New Haven, CT: Yale University Press.

McGoldrick, M., Pearce, J., & Giordano, J. (1982). *Ethnicity and family therapy.* New York: Guilford Press.

Minuchin, S. (1981). *Family therapy techniques.* Cambridge, MA: Harvard University Press.

Wainrib, B. R. (Ed.). (1992). *Gender issues across the life-span.* New York: Springer.

■ ■ ■

6

Parent and Adult Child: Unresolved Issues of Individuation

Albert J. Brok, PhD

A variety of issues emerge between aging parents and adult children; however, there are some intergenerational issues that seem to be typical. One common issue involves the inevitable emotional strain as middle-aged offspring deal with the normal developmental need to continue their own adult individuation and separation from parents. A second issue involves the pressure from parents on single sons and daughters to marry and provide grandchildren. A third issue involves the difficulties aging parents experience in dealing with their own interlife individuation. Often, aging parents displace and rechannel this important later-life developmental task into excessive dependency needs in relation to their offspring. Several other issues exist, such as the need to reconcile different value systems, and emotional factors related to economic and other life situations.

The resolution of all these issues involves the ability of parents and their now adult children to gradually and mutually redefine their relationship from "parent–child" to "adult–adult offspring." When this redefinition is achieved, parents and their adult offspring can have enduring, satisfying, and meaningful mutually supportive times.

When it is not achieved, the result is often emptiness, anomie, and bitterness requiring psychological intervention (Bloom, 1988; Brok, 1990; Brok, 1992; Oldham, 1989).

The purpose of this chapter is to examine issues between adult children and their parents that often emerge during the course of psychotherapy. Case examples will illustrate intergenerational issues that inevitably arise as parents and their adult offspring both grow older chronologically but not necessarily psychologically.

The Case of Gene: Parents, Friends, or What?

The changing nature of the emotional-social tie between parent and offspring as they both age and experience social role changes is an important issue. One major role change involves the redefinition of the parent–offspring relationship.

Gene was a 32-year-old man who entered therapy because of difficulties in his marriage. Specifically, he had been under considerable pressure from his wife Mary to deal with what she considered to be his "immature relationship" with his mother. Gene consistently desired spending vacation time and weekends with his mother and her live-in boyfriend (of course offering to include Mary). Gene considered his mother to be a "friend" rather than a "traditional" mother and could see nothing wrong with the four of them going out on a regular basis. He also saw nothing wrong with discussing his sexual problems and marital issues with his mother, rather than with his wife. Gene would often spend time after work at his mother's house since his wife arrived home quite late from her job. He and mother would play piano duets together, do crossword puzzles, and so forth. Mary complained that her husband never once thought about going directly after work and waiting for her to arrive. Gene claimed that Mary was "just possessive and jealous" of this "friendship" with his mother.

Gene's mother, Dora, had a history of adjustment problems. Dora's father had died when she was five. Her mother remarried within 4 months but divorced her second husband after a year of a stormy marriage, and never remarried. Dora grew up as a confidante and friend to her mother. They shared everything to the point of Dora's mother actually moving to the same college town when Dora went away to school. Dora did manage to separate from her mother by precipitously marrying upon graduation, only to discover that her husband was impotent. They adopted Gene 5 years later and divorced 1 year after that. Dora subsequently took up with a series of men, believing, as Gene put it, in an "open house." Gene grew up as a confidant to his mother. At the time he began therapy, Dora was living with a man 8 years older than Gene.

Gene presented himself as an amiable, unruffled man who always looked at the positive side of things and did not like controversy. He singularly disavowed any aggressive feelings or intentions, even in his dreams. His principal defense seemed to be denial, a defensive style that greatly inhibited his ability to understand the impact his tie to his mother had on his marital relationship.

One aspect of Gene's history was especially important in understanding the nature of his presenting problems. Many, if not all, adopted children need to deal with the traumatic information of their adoption. Some adoptees, aided by empathic and mature parents, can work through the trauma and achieve a relatively successful compromise between depression and optimism. Most seem to remain at least somewhat scarred by the trauma. Gene, however, was without the advantage of having understanding, mature parents—just the opposite. When his mother informed Gene at age 6 that he was adopted, she handled it by feeding her adopted son's growing grandiosity by telling him that this made him "very special, unique, and better" than other children. Gene strongly identified with this. When he proudly told other children about this and they made fun of him, he simply thought they were strange. His omnipotence, already so strong, would only become stronger, reinforced by his intrusive, seductive, and illusion-creating adoptive mother, as well as his experiences with various weak and youthful father figures who came and went. Gene never had to deal with the reality of a continuous father figure and did not have to psychologically compete for his mother's attention. His mother remained the main continuity in his life. This served to bury any feeling he might have had concerning the loss of his biological mother and father. Unconsciously, Gene's adopted mother helped him to deny his trauma and used him to compensate for her earlier difficulties. They both were the center of each other's universes.

The trauma of adoption, the subsequent depression, and his underlying rage and fear of growing up were not dealt with by Gene until he entered into a relatively successful therapeutic experience. Through therapy, Gene was able to initiate a reformulation of his relationship with his mother and stabilize his marriage. As a result of her son's change, Dora, who originally wanted to be in "family therapy" with Gene and his wife, entered her own individual counseling. The process of his mother's treatment gave Gene the space he now craved to work on his own individual and marital life. For her part, Dora seemed to be attempting to rechannel interests and to understand the meaning behind her need to be so closely involved with her son. They were both struggling to work at a new mutuality.

In an extreme way, the preceeding case illustrates the importance of mutual readjustment to roles in later life. Gene needed to grow, and his mother needed to let him go. This task, difficult for well-adjusted parents, was nearly impossible for Dora. An aging parent's task is to individuate into the older adult role—with its privileges as well as its poignancies (Brok, 1992; Oldham, 1989). The privileges include the recognition of one's ongoing separateness, the ability to use one's life experience, the achievement of wisdom, and the enjoyment of one's offspring. The poignancies include the awareness of separation from the now fully adult son or daughter. Parents recognize that they may be loved and appreciated by their offspring but that now they are only a partial recipient of the children's energies, most of which are directed to their own careers, spouses, and offspring.

Friendship within the adult–adult offspring context can only occur when this individuation has been successfully completed. Under these circumstances, one's offspring internalize a healthy sense of their parents, insuring for both a valued sense of continuity within the context of individuality. When this new mutuality is not achieved because of previous parent–child pathology, as in the case of Gene and Dora, the normal adult child–aging parent developmental task is arrested and the parent–child relationship remains dependent and reliant on the induction of guilt.

Reciprocal or "Fourth Individuation"

Reciprocal or "fourth individuation" is a relational developmental task that occurs at midlife for offspring and later life for parents. Both parents and offspring need to recognize their mutual separateness in the context of overall adult relatedness. Where there is considerable parent–offspring overinvolvement, therapists need to emphasize the importance of establishing and maintaining adequate emotional boundaries. Although an initial joint consultation may sometimes be appropriate, parent–offspring issues should be dealt with on an individual basis or in separate therapeutic groups. The very manner in which the therapist structures sessions can have an effect on therapeutic outcome. For example, it would have been a collusion to have seen Dora and Gene together to work out their issues.

The concept of reciprocal or "fourth individuation" builds on and extends earlier individuation processes. These are the separation-individuation tasks developmentally negotiated in the first years of parent–child life (Mahler, Pine, & Bergmann, 1975), the adolescent individuation tasks, or second individuation noted by Erikson (1950) and Blos (1967), and a third individuation in midlife, which involves "a process of intrapsychic structural change that centrally relates to the involution and death of one's parents (Oldham, 1989, p. 89). The fourth individuation makes for the final reformulation of the parent–child relationship, giving it a fully adult-adult status marked by sentimental parent–adult child bonds.

The fourth individuation is different from the third individuation in that it is reciprocally defined. It is a task that can only be negotiated through mutually interactive parent–adult offspring awareness. Parent and offspring each recognize the other's role and context, while feeling the sense of continuity provided by the emotional and historical link that keeps them related. It may be that it is the "last of the offspring," the youngest child, who fully activates this transformation in the parent. One recent film, *Nobody's Fool*, (1995) illustrates this process. In this movie the hero acknowledges the need for his adult son to return to his estranged wife and child, instead of remaining with him.

The Case of Sam: Growing Pains

Sam was 60 years old when he began therapy. The middle of seven children, Sam suffered significant losses when he was young. Having lost his mother when he was 8, he and his siblings were left with their father, described as a distant and uninvolved man. Soon after his mother's death, Sam and his brothers and sisters were placed in various foster homes. Sam was shuffled from place to place. When World War II broke out, Sam enlisted in the army. After the war, he went to law school and graduated but did not practice. Instead, he married and bought into a small business financed by his wife. He became a relatively successful small businessman, had two children, and led an outwardly settled life. After some 28 years of marriage, his wife pursued a divorce in order to enter into a live-in lesbian relationship. This left Sam shocked, depressed, and shaken. Sam's marriage had not been content but had existed, at least outwardly, along traditional lines.

A rather dependent and passively hostile man, Sam entered therapy for the first time in his life at the behest of a woman with whom he was then involved. She complained of what she termed "unsuitable and hostile" jokes toward her friends when she and Sam were in social situations. She also complained that he often lacked appropriate empathy, was too needy, and seemed overinvolved with his grown children. Sam dutifully reported all of this in his first session, advising that he did not know if it was true, but he would "give it [therapy] a shot."

In our initial discussions, Sam revealed that he was a recent grandfather and that he had a lot of difficulty accepting this label, as he felt "young and vital" and not ready for 60 or, as he termed it, being an "elder statesman." His remaining unmarried son, a 24-year-old graduate student, lived with Sam in a small urban apartment Sam had taken after his marriage dissolved.

At the time of treatment, Sam's second son was preparing to move from his father's apartment to live with a woman he intended to marry. Sam consciously liked this woman but questioned his son's decision to move on. On the day of the move, Sam reported he had the following dream:

> I was cleaning wax from my ear with a Q-tip because I could not hear well. I began to feel I couldn't do it and began calling for my son. He appeared and did it for me and I felt great.

Sam's dream had many levels to it. The dream reflected Sam's general reticence to listen and communicate with others, including his children. On another level, Sam's dream revealed his concerns in dealing with a major life transition. This involved both his sense of gender identity, as well as ability to individuate into a significant later-life role. His last son was individuating as an adult and leaving, and Sam desperately wanted to hold on to him. On the one hand, his son's departure revived feelings about the father and, on a deeper level, the mother Sam had lost. On the other hand, his son's leaving threatened to destroy Sam's fantasy of being an active, "on the spot" father. It seemed that Sam needed this active paternal status as direct proof of his potency and male gender identity, which had been greatly battered by his wife's choice of a female sexual partner and his earlier life deprivations. To Sam, his feared age-related role of "elder statesman" was being forced on him because he could not control his children's actions. While appropriately taking charge of their own lives, their actions were serving to loosen the structure of Sam's defensive adaptations, thereby exposing him to considerable suppressed and repressed anxiety. These dynamics served to hinder greatly Sam's capacity to accomplish, on his own, the normally difficult but usually manageable task of later-life individuation from one's children. Instead, his dependency needs in relation to his last offspring had remained paramount.

The early death of Sam's mother and his father's subsequent abdication of his parental role had left Sam feeling abandoned and vulnerable, his rageful anger being handled by various defensive maneuvers. His wife's leaving and his son's adult individuation were used in the therapeutic setting to help Sam rework past conflicts. This, in turn, allowed him to work on current life stage normative transitions and age-relevant roles such as grandfather, father-in-law, and father–adult son relationships. Both Sam and his son were able to mutually and reciprocally deal with their respective life tasks.

The Case of Selma: Mourning the Past

Selma came into treatment at age 38. She had moved out of her parental home only 6 months earlier and was feeling depressed, anxious, and lonely. She dated infrequently and was a virgin. Her sexual experience had been limited to some light kissing when she was in college.

A significant factor of Selma's family history was that her parents were both severely traumatized Holocaust survivors. Both her mother and father had lost all their relatives in German concentration camps during World War II. Selma's father survived by passing himself off as a Christian after escaping from a work camp in Poland. He lived day to day in fear of being found out for almost 4 years. At work he could not even go to the toilet when there were other men present out of fear someone would see his circumcised penis and report him as a Jew. He had personally seen his parents taken off to concentration camps, while he was kept behind with a labor squad. He never saw them or his other relatives again. Selma's mother had survived the war in a concentration camp. She, too, had lost all her relatives including parents, four sisters, and two brothers.

Selma's parents met in a displaced persons camp after the war and quickly married when they found out they were from the same city. Their marriage, while lasting through the present, was clearly initiated out of desperation to hang on to something familiar. They moved to Israel and then to the United States. Selma was their only child. She grew up with no extended family and without a picture of her grandparents or other relatives. She and her parents lived essentially as one, forming a tight little community. Selma had individuated to some extent by going away to college; however, she returned home immediately after graduation. Although she earned a substantially good income during the next 17 years, she did not leave home to live on her own until she was 38.

Both parents related to Selma as the fantasied reincarnation of their respective parents, particularly their mothers. Selma's father did this overtly by naming his daughter after his mother (without consulting his wife). More covertly, his overinvolvement with his daughter was abetted by his strong dependency needs and latent Oedipally tinged drives, which underlay his relationship with her. For example, as Selma blossomed into adolescence, she and her father would go out to the movies three Saturday nights a month, while mother stayed home, because mother "didn't enjoy films." After Selma moved out, her father would call her every morning to make sure she woke up on time and would come to spend the day with her on Sunday. Selma did not object to this until she began to realize in therapy how this was stifling her own independence and how guilty she was about being "disloyal" to her father's need to have her live out a projection of his lost mother.

This is a somewhat common dynamic existing between parents and children. Often parents have difficulty individuating and separating into their own adulthood because they have not been able to grieve and mourn the loss (real or emotional) of their own parents. Wishes for one's lost parent are often projected onto children, who are then induced to unconsciously play out that role. This is one of the bases for "parentified" children. When parents have been traumatized, the issue is even more powerful than in less extreme situations (Pines, 1986).

Selma's mother, of course, colluded with the mutually symbiotic father–daughter relationship. A rather distant, "numbed" woman, she was ambivalently attached to her husband and daughter. Her need to relate did not go much beyond being with her family in a distant way. She did not crave privacy with her husband. For example, when the family would go on vacation, all three would sleep in the same hotel room, "to save money," even though they had adequate funds for separate rooms.

Selma's entry into therapy, itself a step toward individuation, not only helped her personally develop and reformulate her conscious and unconscious relation with her parents, but it also forced her parents to deal with the change in her and thus with their own life situation. Selma was able to free herself from her unconscious identification with her parents' need to have Selma be their parents (parents who would never abandon them!). She was able to successfuly deal with the intense sense of disloyalty she felt in living her own life and realized that she was not betraying or abandoning her parents by moving out into the world. (Her parents had unconsciously equated moving out with going to near-certain death in a concentration camp.)

With Selma's continued separation and subsequent individuation from them acting as a catalyst, her parents slowly, partially, and painfully mourned the loss of their own parents. This freedom enabled them to go on a vacation trip alone for the first time in their lives. Selma, through her risk of confronting her parents with her need for autonomy, risked her anxiety that this disloyalty would lead to their demise.

In short, a change in one part of the parent–adult child system (Selma) changed the basis for the whole system, in this case for the better. Selma began dating. She had also learned much about her parents' history, a history they had not shared out of their need to keep her protected from a "harsh, cruel world." In part, her parents' protectiveness was a way of keeping the fantasy alive that their parents were not really gone, but lived on in Selma.

Summary

Relations between parents and adult offspring are complex. A significant task is for both parties to come to terms with the individual trajectory of their respective lives. The term *fourth individuation* highlights a significant intergenerational task that can only be resolved mutually and reciprocally. When this later-life developmental task is not achieved, blunted development and stagnation for both parties occurs. The cases of Gene, Sam, and Selma and their respective familial issues illustrate how appropriate therapeutic intervention can transform a stunted parent–child system into a healthy adult–adult offspring relationship.

References

Bloom, M. V. (1988). Leaving home: A family transition. In J. Bloom-Feschbach & S. Bloom-Feschbach (Eds.), *The psychology of separation and loss* (pp. 232–266). San Francisco: Jossey-Bass.

Blos, P. (1967). The second individuation process of adolescence. In R. Eissler, A. Freud, & M. Kris (Eds.), *The psychoanalytic study of the child*, (Vol. 22, pp. 162–186). New York: International Universities Press.

Brok, A. J. (1990, March). *Understanding stage of life issues and genetic conflicts with late-life patients*. Paper presented at the Mid-Winter

Convention, Division 29 (Psychotherapy) of the American Psychological Association, Palm Springs, CA.

Brok, A. J. (1992). Crises and transitions: Gender and life stage issues in individual, group, and couples treatment. *Psychoanalysis and Psychotherapy, 10*, 3–16.

Erikson, E. (1950). *Childhood and society.* New York: Norton.

Mahler, M., Pine, F., & Bergmann, A. (1975). *The psychological birth of the human infant.* New York: Basic Books.

Oldham, J. M. (1989). The third individuation, middle-aged children and their parents. In J. M. Oldham & R. S. Liebert (Eds.), *The middle years* (pp. 89–104). New Haven, CT: Yale University Press.

Pines, D. (1986). Working with women survivors of the Holocaust: Affective experiences in transference and countertransference. *International Journal of Psychoanalysis, 67*, 295–307.

■ ■ ■

7

Missing Fathers: Aging Traditional Men and Familial Estrangement

Gary R. Brooks, PhD

For decades, family therapists have expressed concern about missing or "peripheral" fathers, men who are either emotionally or physically unavailable to their children (Brooks & Gilbert, 1995; Brooks & Silverstein, 1995; Silverstein, 1993). If this lack of availability were conceptualized along a continuum, at one end would be fathers who have minimal emotional involvement, although they are physically present in the home. At the other end would be those fathers who are not only emotionally absent but also are rarely or never seen by their children.

Family therapists have shown considerable concern about the first situation, in which fathers not only refuse to participate in therapy but also exert a restraining influence on the entire process. Doherty (1981) stated that "involving the reluctant father is one of the central practical issues in family sessions" (p. 23).

Many family therapy leaders have long seen the participation of fathers as pivotal to treatment. Whitaker (1973, p. 3) stated, "If you don't seduce the father in the first interview, you've had it." Kaslow (1981) noted that a father's participation is "essential." The research of Shapiro and Budman (1973, p. 58) found that "a father's attitude toward treatment is critical in determining whether a family remains in treatment—unless the father is positively involved the treatment is likely to fail."

Although the attention to fathers' participation has, according to feminist family therapists (Avis, 1988; Bograd, 1991), sometimes reached inappropriate levels, the frequency of this complaint certainly reflects the extent of concern about men's emotional disconnection.

The more extreme position on this continuum of disconnection—fathers' emotional and physical absence from the home—has also been a major concern of social scientists over the years.

In his review of American fathering, Pleck (1987) described the period of 1940–1965 as one in which there was great concern about the unavailability of fathers as role models for children, especially sons. At that time, the predominant developmental theory held that "male identity is thwarted by boys' initial identification with their mothers and by high rates of father absence" (Pleck, 1987, p. 92) As this theory evolved, fathers were also seen as essential for healthy development of daughters. According to Pleck, this developmental theory of father-as-sex-role-model has been superseded by a "new father" model, one that has been enriched by the work of Chodorow (1978), Dinnerstein (1976), Levant (1992), and Silverstein (1993). Although this newer theory revises much earlier thinking, father involvement continues to be a major concern of family observers. Silverstein (1993) stated, "If men do not change there is little hope for lasting change in women and children....Redefining fathering has the potential to transform society" (p. 282).

Because of their concern about absent fathers, family therapists have expended considerable energy not only in trying to increase fathers' participation in their families but also in theorizing about the causes of fathers' uninvolvement. Although a great deal may be learned by studying the father-absent family, a different body of information might be acquired through a more direct approach—studying the absent father himself.

How would these men themselves explain their experiences of isolation from their children? Answering this question is difficult, because troubled men frequently avoid psychologists' offices (Scher, 1990; Vessey & Howard, 1993). Instead of seeking professional help, men are likely to adopt a variety of maladaptive coping techniques to reduce psychic distress—substance abuse, violence, emotional isolation, and flight. Though not commonly found in psychologists' offices, troubled traditional men are often found in institutional settings—homeless shelters, alcohol halfway houses, prisons, and

VA domiciliaries ("old soldiers homes")—where they might be studied. What can be learned about traditional men's estrangement through interviews with men in these settings?

The material that follows is based on my clinical experiences in a VA domiciliary, with a population of traditional men, many of whom have been estranged from their children for many years. A case example is presented to illustrate some of the issues. Although no empirical research has been conducted, numerous interviews with these men have helped generate hypotheses regarding factors contributing to their physical and emotional isolation. This chapter concludes with implications for therapists.

An Estranged Father

Henry, a 57-year-old African American retired army sergeant, was referred to Psychology Service as part of his processing for domiciliary admission. Henry had a 20-year history of alcohol abuse, though he had had 8 years of sobriety working as an alcohol rehabilitation counselor. Several months before coming to the VA, he had returned to the use of alcohol. When initially interviewed, he was noted to be sad, remorseful, and "emotionally empty." Two weeks later, he was reinterviewed to explore the factors in his life that may have led to his estrangement from his family.

Henry had married his wife Marie when both were teenagers and Henry was approaching army enlistment. Within the next 10 years they had three daughters and one son. As part of his military career, Henry was often absent from the home, sometimes for many months. Marie was a homemaker and frequently was forced to function as a single parent. Despite the separations, Henry was able to speak proudly about his ability to "provide" for his family and about the fact that the children had received good educations. In his words, "Back then it wasn't exactly easy for Black families in the South."

After Henry's army retirement, the couple experienced considerable interpersonal conflict. Henry's alcohol use increased. Marie sought a divorce. Of this, Henry said "I was totally shocked that she did that." Henry left the geographical area and "threw himself into the bottle." Over the next several years, he lost all contact with his children. He heard nothing about them until a few weeks before hospital admission when his son visited, found him seriously ill, and brought him to the VA.

When asked to talk about his loss of connection with his children, Henry became quite emotional. His voice dropped to a low volume and his eyes teared. He spoke slowly, with several pauses. He emphasized his satisfaction that the children had grown up without major problems and that he had been a decent financial provider. "I always saw that they had what they needed, even when I couldn't be there for them." He went on, however, to express great remorse about what he had not participated in, about the "family times" that would never take place again.

When asked to try to come up with reasons for his years of disconnection from the children, he cited several factors.

First, he expressed shame about his heavy alcohol use and his "rejection" by his wife. He said that when he served in Vietnam, he had been "classified as some kind of hero for saving two guys' lives." He was deeply attached to that war-hero role, as he felt that it was a major source of his children's respect for him. Sadly, he felt that his children needed to have "a high image of me.... It would hurt them to see who I really am and how I feel." Henry was gratified that he had been able to keep his children from seeing him during his "worst periods of drunkedness."

Related to Henry's need to perpetuate a war-hero image was a theme about his difficulty with emotional interdependence. He said, "I always wanted to provide for my children.... I didn't want to ask them for anything." Even during the most intensely painful portions of the postdivorce period, Henry never allowed himself to seek the emotional support of his children, partially because he feared their censure or rejection.

A third factor in Henry's avoidance of his children was his inability to tolerate rekindling of powerful melancholic memories and his grief about missed opportunities for closer attachments. Instead of exposing himself to these sources of pain, he attempted to insulate himself through alcohol use and geographical distancing.

Finally, Henry's description of the family environment suggested that of the many family symptom patterns, his alcohol use was a major one in stabilizing family tension—as long as he was drinking and unavailable, a degree of family equilibrium was possible (at great expense to all).

Traditional Masculinity and Familial Estrangement

Henry's case illustrates several themes in masculine socialization that may contribute to the absence of fathers from their families.

Constricted Father Roles

The traditional role of father has emphasized breadwinner and leadership functions, with little value placed on caretaking and nurturing (Levant & Kelly, 1989; Pleck, 1987). Historically, men have measured each other according to their achievements in the world of work, not in the world of nurturing babies and guiding children. Young men are typically discouraged from entering situations where child care skills can be developed. Furthermore, many of the skills and personal attributes that facilitate good parenting—sensitivity, communication skills, acceptance of vulnerability—are among those that are usually considered "unmasculine."

The breadwinner role, the central aspect of most men's identity, typically requires men to be so work-focused that parenting and nurturing are given a far lower priority. Part of the problem, of course, is the high degree of demand that work places on men's physical and emotional energies. Equally important, however, is the low status men ascribe to childcare and men's common lack of competence in many childcare skills (Levant, 1994; Levant & Kelly, 1989).

The Big Wheel

David and Brannon's (1976) description of the male role emphasized men's need to be seen as successful, competent, and accomplished persons: the "big wheel." Masculinity is not a given, but an achieved status, sought through continual competition with other men for the appearance of success. In the words of Willie Loman in *Death of a Salesman*, "A man can't go out in the way he came in, Ben, a man has got to add up to something" (Miller, 1956, p. 286).

This need to achieve "big wheel" status provides a sense of purpose to men's lives but may also generate considerable insecurity. Men who fail are subject to being viewed as losers. Even if men are able to reach "big wheel" status, they are still prone to rate themselves negatively in relation to "bigger wheels." Worse, if they encounter a significant drop in status through disability, unemployment, or retirement, they often experience devastating emotional crises.

A particularly unfortunate aspect of this phenomenon is that unrealistic images of masculinity pressure men to "stay in charge" of the family, making it most difficult to cope with their children's increasing autonomy (or with a spouse's push for empowerment).

With Henry, we saw painful evidence of how the need to be a "big wheel," to protect his self-image of heroism, kept him from an authentic connection with his children. Family therapy could have helped

Henry and the children free themselves from the needs and fanta-
sies of the past—to see Henry in a more realistic and forgiving light.

No Sissy Stuff—The Sturdy Oak

Other dimensions of the masculine role noted by David and
Brannon (1976), "No Sissy Stuff" and "The Sturdy Oak," are additional factors that may contribute to fathers' estrangement from
their children.

From an early age, men are taught to avoid anything viewed as
"feminine," especially interpersonal sensitivity and the expression
of tender emotions. Affection for children is more easily demonstrated through financial contributions and career self-sacrifice than
through sharing of intimate moments or emotional availability during life crises. The delegation of affective and nurturing functions
to mothers often produces alienation of fathers from the most intense connections with children.

Further perpetuating this emotional distancing is the need men
often feel to appear tough, confident, and self-reliant, to live up to
the "sturdy oak" dictate of the male role. Just as "no sissy stuff"
deprives men of access to children's pain, the "sturdy oak" man-
date deprives them of the opportunity to receive children's emotional support. Oftentimes, in an effort to maintain an emotionally
tough image during a time of personal distress, men will avoid intimacy through withdrawal, denial, or flight, sometimes coupled with
alcohol or substance abuse.

Substance Abuse

Men are four to five times more likely than women to abuse alcohol (Gomberg, 1979). Many factors may predispose men to adopt
alcohol abuse as a coping mechanism, such as socialized messages
about manliness and alcohol, difficulties with emotional expressiveness, intolerance of certain negative affects (grief and guilt), or
biological susceptibility to addiction. Whatever the precipitant, once
a pattern of alcohol abuse has begun, a reciprocal process of familial estrangement typically follows: He drinks because he is alienated and rejected; he is alienated and rejected because he drinks.

Violence

Fasteau (1975, p. 149) called violence the "crucible of manhood."
Men are given highly contradictory messages about violence, from

glorification to vilification. The ambiguity of messages given to men about violence, coupled with another feature of male socialization—emotional inexpressiveness—create a potent environment for men's familial estrangement.

Men's problems with emotional expressiveness, well described by Balswick (1988) and Levant (1994), generally do not extend to difficulties with expression of anger. Traditional men are quick to experience and express anger. In fact, the conceptualization of the "male emotional funnel system" (Long, 1987, p. 310) identifies a tendency for men to channel all their painful affect into the experiencing of anger.

Intense and poorly modulated anger can frequently lead to interpersonal violence. Once initiated, violence, like alcohol abuse, may become part of a reciprocal cycle producing a man's estrangement.

Because of the enormous physical and emotional suffering resulting from men's violence, most therapists, not surprisingly, have primarily focused their attentions on the plight of the victims. Less obvious are the long-term effects of this violence on many of the perpetrators. My interviews with formerly violent men, many years after separation from families, sometimes yield an interesting finding. Some of these men, anguished over the pain they inflicted, have voluntarily chosen to isolate themselves from their families, rather than risk further harm to loved ones. Several have told me, "I'd rather kill myself than hurt my family any further."

No claim is being made that these men are representative of the "batterer" population. Instead, I report this observation only to illustrate how violence, an integral feature of traditional male socialization, can sometimes be one of the factors that contributes to a man's familial isolation.

Blocked Life Cycle Development

From the observations of Jung (1960) to the empirical research of Neugarten and Guttman (1958) and Vaillant (1994), a commonly accepted belief has developed that men become more "nurturant and other-centered" as they age. "It has been frequently stated that the older American man becomes either more androgynous or more feminized over time" (Solomon, 1982, p. 208). This feminization phenomenon could be good news for those concerned about peripheral fathers. If true, men, after many years of establishing themselves as "masculine" persons, would then shift, albeit belatedly, to give greater attention to the nurturing of children. Unfortunately, this belief has had only mixed empirical support (Solomon, 1982). Additionally, this idea seems to have a pronounced element of class bias.

In a paper that reviewed the popular models of men's life span development, Moreland (1980) proposed that at midlife, men should be able to move beyond "adolescent" models of masculinity (i.e., masculinity characteristic of traditional men). The key to this transformation would be a shift in emphasis from "physical strength and prowess to emphasis on a combination of intellectual and interpersonal skills...particularly in terms of more mutually satisfying relationships with women" (p. 813). Men making this transition would be open to greater interpersonal sensitivity, more expression of vulnerability, and less emphasis on competition; in short, they could become more emotionally responsive husbands and fathers. "Men can become more nurturant to their primary partners and their children since they now view them less as extensions of their achieving striving selves, and more as individuals in their own right" (Moreland, 1980, p. 816).

Unfortunately, this growth model of male development, with its optimistic suggestions that men make their mark and then relax, seems quite out of touch with the realities of life for many blue-collar traditional men. Among this group of men there rarely is a sense of having made one's mark or of being able to leave the world of physical challenge and danger (Lazur & Majors, 1995; Rubin, 1976). According to Shostak (1972, p. 4), the "macho" role expectations for "controlling one's spouse, sexual conquest, and authoritarian rule in the home" vary little throughout the life cycle.

From the classic writings of Jung (1960) and Erickson (1980) to the more recent work of Levinson, Darrow, Klein, Levinson, and McKee (1978) and Thompson (1994), most writing about the man's life cycle development suggests a gradual "feminizing." That is, most theorists believe that men, as they age successfully, broaden their masculine gender role to include elements formerly thought unmasculine (tenderness, compassion, and more nurturing connections with others). Unfortunately, many working-class men like Henry are impeded in this process, partially because of their continual struggles in establishing even the most rudimentary sense of life accomplishment. As a result, while some men move toward nurturance, many others struggle with pressures that perpetuate family estrangement.

Implications for Therapists

The preceding material has demonstrated trends in the socialization of traditional men that may contribute to familial estrangement. Based on these observations, a number of clinical implications seem worthy of consideration.

Gender Sensitive Family Therapy

Familial estrangement of traditional men, when conceptualized as an outgrowth of male socialization, cannot be adequately confronted without gender sensitive interventions. As I have argued previously (Brooks, 1990), family therapists must have a deep appreciation of the socialization experiences of all family members. In the special situation of estranged fathers, therapists must understand how traditional male role pressures cause men to seek emotional withdrawal or geographic distance from their children.

Collusion To Omit Men From Therapy

Fathers' absence from family therapy sessions will continue to be a problem as long as that absence seems to provide equilibrium for the family system, emotional benefits for the withdrawing male, and greater comfort for the family therapist. The feminist objection that fathers should not be patronized or idealized in efforts to secure participation (Bograd, 1986, 1991) seems appropriate.

Nevertheless, therapists should not give up too quickly. Earnest efforts should be made to connect with men in a manner that is likely to succeed. Sometimes, separate meetings with the father may be helpful to discuss his perspective. Therapists familiar with the coping style and role pressures of traditional men have an improved chance of making an initial connection with these men and of demonstrating that therapy could be beneficial for them.

Possibilities For Reconnection

Those therapists working in settings with male populations should be aware of opportunities to reconnect estranged fathers with their children. Though few traditional men will spontaneously request efforts to reconnect with children as a major therapy objective, therapists should be alert for signs of interest. Of course, this is an enormously complex issue in which the needs, interests, emotional well-being, and physical safety of all family members must be weighed carefully.

Despite the complications, therapists must give greater emphasis to fathers' reconnection with children. Sometimes a modest objective, such as helping an estranged father find a way to become comfortable with resumption of financial commitment to his children, may help provide a man with substantial emotional benefits.

New Models of Fathering

A major factor causing men to flee from their families is their conviction that only certain types of family contributions are worthy of fathers. When men learn to broaden their definitions of fatherhood to include companionship, nurturing, and emotionally supportive roles, they will have less need to be preoccupied with the traditionally narrow roles. Sometimes, painful losses such as unemployment, retirement, or physical disability can be used to promote greater involvement in fathering. A skillful therapist can help these men recognize that their new nonworker status, although a significant loss, is also a new golden opportunity to father (or grandfather). Although retirement, unemployment, or disabilty will always pose a major adjustment challenge, they may be seen to have at least one silver lining—a fresh opportunity to become engrossed in the lives of children and loved ones.

Male Self-Discovery and Emotional Skills

Men's estrangement from families will be lessened when men become more facile at managing their affective lives without resorting to extreme and alienating behaviors, such as alcohol use, violence, or flight. It is useful to provide men with psychoeducational activities that emphasize emotional expressiveness, assertiveness, and anger management. Additionally, because many men are grossly unaware of how gender role socialization contributes to their psychosocial stresses, men can benefit greatly from participation in male consciousness-raising activities.

Summary

For many years family therapists have been concerned about peripheral or missing fathers. Although, in most cases, fathers have certainly been "present" in terms of their financial contributions and willingness to sacrifice their health for the good of their families, they have often been "absent" from many of the richly rewarding affective family experiences. In some more unfortunate instances, men have not only been affectively marginal, they have also been physically absent. The estrangement of traditional men from their children is deeply rooted in male socialization. Family therapists are in a unique position to help these men and their families. Gender sensitive family therapists can empathize with the gender role pressures of all family members, thereby helping men develop new concepts of fathering, reconnect with their children, and end their isolation from their families.

References

Avis, J. M. (1988). Deepening awareness: A private study guide to feminism and family therapy. In L. Braverman (Ed.), *A guide to feminist family therapy* (pp. 15–46). New York: Harrington Park.

Balswick, J. O. (1988). *The inexpressive male.* Lexington, MA: Lexington Books.

Bograd, M. (1986). A feminist examination of family systems models of violence against women in the family. In M. Ault-Riché (Ed.), *Women in family therapy* (pp. 34–50). Rockville, MD: Aspen Systems.

Bograd, M. (Ed.). (1991). *Feminist approaches for men in family therapy.* New York: Haworth Press.

Brooks, G. R. (1990). Psychotherapy with traditional role oriented males. In P. A. Keller & L. G. Ritt (Eds.), *Innovations in clinical practice: A source book* (pp. 61–74). Sarasota, FL: Professional Resource Exchange.

Brooks, G. R., & Gilbert, L. A. (1995). Men in families: Old constraints, new possibilities. In R. F. Levant & W. S. Pollack (Eds.), *A new psychology of men* (pp. 252–279). New York: Basic Books.

Brooks, G. R., & Silverstein, L. B. (1995). Understanding the dark side of masculinity: An integrative systems model. In R. F. Levant & W. S. Pollack (Eds.), *A new psychology of men* (pp. 280–336). New York: Basic Books.

Chodorow, N. (1978). *The reproduction of mothering.* Berkeley: University of California Press.

David, D. S., & Brannon, R. (1976). *The forty-nine percent majority: The male sex role.* Reading, MA: Addison-Wesley.

Dinnerstein, D. (1976). *The mermaid and the minotaur: Sexual arrangements and human malaise.* New York: Harper & Row.

Doherty, W. J. (1981). Involving the reluctant father in family therapy. In A. S. Gurman (Ed.), *Questions and answers in the practice of family therapy* (pp. 23–26). New York: Brunner/Mazel.

Erickson, E. (1980). *Identity and the life cycle.* New York: Norton.

Fasteau, M. F. (1975). *The male machine.* New York: Dell.

Gomberg, E. S. (1979). Problems with alcohol and other drugs. In E. S. Gomberg & V. Franks (Eds.), *Gender and disordered behavior: Sex differences in psychopathology* (pp. 204–240). New York: Brunner/Mazel.

Jung, C. G. (1960). The structure and dynamics of the psyche. In *Collected works* (Vol. 8). Princeton, NJ: Princeton University Press.

Kaslow, F. W. (1981). Involving the peripheral father in family therapy. In
A. S. Gurman (Ed.), *Questions and answers in the practice of family
therapy* (pp. 27–31). New York: Brunner/Mazel.

Lazur, R. F., & Majors, R. (1995). Men of color: Ethnocultural variations of
male gender role strain. In R. F. Levant & W. S. Pollack (Eds.), *A new
psychology of men* (pp 337–358). New York: Basic Books.

Levant, R. (1992). Toward the reconstruction of masculinity. *Journal of
Family Psychology, 5,* 379–402.

Levant, R. F. (1994). *Masculinity reconstructed: Changing the rules of manhood—at work, in relationships, and in family life.* New York: Dutton.

Levant. R., & Kelley, J. (1989). *Between father and child.* New York: Vi-
king.

Levinson, D. J., Darrow, C. N., Klein, E. B., Levinson, M. H., & McKee, B.
(1978). *The seasons of a man's life.* New York: Knopf.

Long, D. (1987). Working with men who batter. In M. Scher, M. Stevens, G.
Good, & G. Eichenfield (Eds.), *Handbook of counseling and psychotherapy with men* (pp. 305–320). Newbury Park, CA: Sage.

Miller, A. (1956). *Death of a salesman.* In E. B. Watson & B. Pressey (Eds.),
Contemporary drama: Eleven plays. New York: Scribner.

Moreland, J. (1980). Age and change in the adult male sex role. *Sex Roles,
6,* 807–818.

Neugarten, B., & Guttman, D. (1958). Age-sex roles and personality in middle
age: A thematic apperception study. *Psychological Monographs, 470,*
1–33.

Pleck, J. H. (1987). American fathering in historical perspective. In M. S.
Kimmel (Ed.), *Changing men: New directions in research on men
and masculinity* (pp. 83–97). Beverly Hills, CA: Sage.

Rubin, L. B. (1976). *Worlds of pain: Life in the working class family.*
New York: Basic Books.

Scher, M. (1990). Effect of gender-role incongruities on men's experience
as clients in psychotherapy. *Psychotherapy, 27,* 322–326.

Shapiro, R. J., & Budman, S. H. (1973). Defection, termination, and continuation in family therapy. *Family Process, 12,* 55–67.

Shostak, A. (1972). Middle-aged working class Americans at home. *Occu-
pational Mental Health, 3,* 2–7.

Silverstein, L. (1993). Primate research, family politics, and social policy.
Transforming "cads" into "dads." *Journal of Family Psychology, 7,* 267–
282.

Solomon, K. (1982). The older man. In K. Solomon & N. Levy (Eds.), *Men
in transition: Theory and therapy* (pp. 205–240). New York: Plenum.

Thompson, E. H. (1994). *Older men's lives.* Thousands Oaks, CA: Sage.

Vaillant, G. E. (1994). "Successful again" and psychosocial well-being:
Evidence from a 45 year study. In E. H. Thompson (Ed.), *Older men's
lives* (pp. 22–41). Thousand Oaks, CA: Sage.

Vessey, J. T., & Howard, K. I. (1993). Who seeks psychotherapy? *Psychotherapy, 30,* 546–553.

Whitaker, C. (1973). *The technique of family therapy.* Ackerman Memorial Address, Family Institute of Philadelphia Annual Conference, Philadelphia, PA.

■ ■ ■

8

When Golden Pond is Tainted: Domestic Violence and the Elderly

Irene Deitch, PhD

"MURDER ENDS LIFETIME TOGETHER....Man, 75, Accused of Strangling Wife, 72....Motives Remain Unclear" (*Staten Island Advance*, July 1993)

"Son chains mother to the bed and locks the door to the room. Although she is 'fed' she is restrained from responding to phone calls and is beaten when she cries." (National Aging Resource Center on Elder Abuse video)

T he elderly are the fastest growing segment of the population (Tatara, 1991, 1993; Tomes, 1993). With the death rate slowing down, the population of the oldest-old will explode. Currently, 13,000 people are over the age of 100. The majority of this group are women. Life span increases because those persons entering older age are generally healthier.

Family abuse of elders is one of the most neglected areas in the study of family psychology (Tatara, 1990). Hudson (1991) described the harmful consequences of destructive behavior occurring within a family relationship. Attention must be directed to those circumstances within couple and family systems that may predictably predispose family members to abusive behaviors (Steinmetz, 1988; Wolf, 1992).

Although the goal of this chapter is to sensitize family counselors to those family members who are violating the quality of life of their elderly, we must not be misled by the myth that families of older people are uncaring, unconcerned, and unavailable and therefore unfit to serve as surrogate decision makers. Even though 80% of caregiving is performed by family members, usually adult children or spouses, and only 5% of the elderly are institutionalized, there exists an antifamily trend (Hugh, 1991; Pritchard, 1993).

Unfortunately, though, abuse does exist. The 200,000 cases of reported elder abuse do not accurately reflect the extent of the problem. It is estimated that only 1 out of 14 cases of abuse is reported to the authorities. Most victims are reluctant to report the abuser, because most forms of abuse occur within the home and by family members. A more accurate estimate is 2 million incidents (National Aging Resource Center on Elder Abuse, 1990; Stein, 1991; Tatara,1993). The Shiferaw and Mittlemark (1994) study of abuse statistics found that a majority of cases involved victims aged 75 and older, with 70% of victims being women and 63% White. Among the cases of substantiated physical abuse, the abuser was most often a spouse, followed by an adult child or grandchild (New York City Department for the Aging, 1990).

Sex and gender play a significant but often unrecognized role in domestic violence against elderly women (Deitch, 1994; Ramsey-Klawsnik, 1993; Sengstock, 1991; Tallmer, 1996). In a Washington news conference (May 5, 1994), the Older Women's League reported statistics indicating that the murder rate for women aged 65 and older rose 30% since 1974, while the murder rate for men the same age declined 6%. In 1991, 40% of crimes against women aged 65 and older were committed by family members, friends, or acquaintances. Clearly, elder abuse is a women's issue!

Although violence is regarded as a major public health issue in the United States, the elderly are generally excluded as the focus of research in family violence. Several hypotheses are presented to describe the etiology and dynamics of elder abuse. Family therapists need to understand that multiple approaches are necessary in addressing these issues. In this chapter, a working framework is offered in which gender, ethnic differences, cultural differences, psychopathology, clinical gerontology, and family dynamics are used to assess the abusers, why their victims are reluctant to seek assistance, and why victims remain in abusive situations. Biases against the elderly (ageism), along with misinformation and myths related to the developmental aspects of aging, are shown to contribute to the relative neglect of this area of study. According to Tatara (1990), elder abuse is anticipated to be the problem of the next century.

Drawing on psychopathology, psychotherapy, and feminist studies, this chapter uses a family violence framework. Developmental and clinical issues of later adulthood are described to help counselors understand the issues of the aging family member. Abuse prevention, recognition, and intervention strategies by therapists are explored. Directions for further research and policy recommendations with implications for family psychology are discussed.

Background

The introduction of the phrase "granny battering" raised the public's awareness and led to disclosures of a previously hidden problem. This increase in attention and reporting parallels the acknowledgement of incidents of child battering, wife battering, incest, sexual abuse, and rape (Utech & Garrett, 1992). However, applying a child battering model to understanding the nature of elder abuse helps to perpetuate stereotypical perceptions of the elderly as helpless, fragile, dependent, and childlike. Research on elderly victimization lags far behind the research on child and spousal abuse.

The application of research from the fields of gerontology, family systems, and family violence is also neglected in studying elder abuse. Sensationalistic media reports reinforce erroneous assumptions that "aging" is the cause of victimization. Distortions of the elderly as demented, debilitated, and diseased lead to greater concern for the caregiving family member. The caregiver's burden and stresses, as a consequence of the care recipient's physical and emotional dependence, are also thought to have caused the abuse and have resulted in "blaming the victim for the abusive situation" (Parks & Pilisuk, 1991; Petel, Casserta, Hutton, & Lund, 1988; Pillemer & Finkelhor, 1988, 1989; Simon, 1992).

In seeking other explanations for elder mistreatment by family members, there emerges a profile: "the woman in the middle." She is usually described as the adult daughter or daughter-in-law, trapped by familial obligations, faced with overwhelming demands of caregiving and the competing pressures of her family of conception and work responsibilities (Petel et al., 1988). Pillemer and Suitor's (1989, 1991) research focused on whether this type of caregiver is more vulnerable to acting out frustrations, thereby creating an abusive situation.

Another explanation for elder abuse suggests that the abusive parent might become the abused elderly. Using child abuse and spouse abuse as models, elder abuse is believed to be related to the "cycle of violence" theory (Pillemer & Finkelhor, 1989; Pillemer & Suitor, 1989).

Methodological approaches used to study domestic abuse of the elderly have proven somewhat limited in attempts to apply the results of the studies to diverse minority and cultural groups (Stein, 1991; Wolf, 1994). Currently, agencies, educational institutions, and organizations on local, state, and national levels are interfacing to design projects and programs to support research and to train and educate the public and professionals in the recognition, assessment, and treatment of the elderly victims and their families.

Nature of Elder Abuse

Aging parents represent a diverse population. Although some are frail, ill or disabled, widowed or uncoupled, others are active and autonomous. Frequently these older parents are caregivers to their elderly parents, their spouses, or their dependent adult children (Greenberg, Seltzer, & Greenley, 1993; Troll, 1993). The aging parent can be romantically involved and continue to be sexually responsive, challenging the myth of the asexual older person (Tallmer, 1996).

In their study of elder abuse in Boston, Pillemer and Finkelhor (1988) found abuse to be prevalent in more than 3% of the population of persons over 65, a statistic disputed by Tatara (1993), whose data reflected a higher incidence. Spousal abuse was found to occur more frequently than abuse by adult children (New York City Department for the Aging, 1991; Pillemer & Finkelhor, 1989; Sengstock, 1991). The prohibition of adult child against parental abuse is stronger than that of spouse to spouse abuse (Hwalek, Quinn, & Goodrich, 1993). The majority of the elders who are the abused are described as Caucasian, female, widowed, and between the ages of 60 and 85. If the abuser is married to the victim and an informal caregiver, intervention is more likely to be successful.

The physical and emotional dependency of the victim as reasons for familial abuse were disputed by Pillemer and Finkelhor (1989). Their case-controlled research did not support either caregiver stress or care recipient's physical status as a basis for abuse. Significant variables for the abusive behaviors were abuser deviance and dependency. These findings are consistent with those of family violence research, which shows that abuser characteristics are more significant predictors of violence than are victim characteristics. Pillemer and Finkelhor (1989) found that abusers have more mental, emotional, alcohol, and drug related problems and tend to be more dependent on their victims. The abuser was often found to be a cognitively impaired or mentally ill adult child, spouse, or grandchild who was dependent on the aged parent or grandparent (Anetzberger, 1987; Pillemer & Finkelhor, 1989). Abuser deviance was also cited as a most predictive variable of violence (Breckman & Adelman, 1988; Pillemer, 1985; Sukosky, 1992).

Other contributing factors to domestic violence against the elderly are social isolation of the family, reverse spousal abuse (Sengstock, 1991), and victim pathology (i.e., Alzheimer's disease and dementia; Pillemer & Suitor, 1989). Paveza et al. (1992) found that out of the 17% general prevalence of violence in the caregiving patient situation, 4% of the families caregiving the Alzheimer patient were abusive. Caregiver depression and living arrangement with the immediate family were predictive of the abuse. Wolf (1995), comparing prevalence studies of elder abuse in families with those families having Alzheimer's patients, suggested that the risk of abuse in families with an Alzheimer's patient may be greater than that found in a general population sample.

Models for Understanding Domestic Elder Abuse

Gerontological Model

Aging is not a disease, nor is it the cause of violence. Stereotypes of the elderly as "functionally incapacitated" (Troll, 1993) or sexually inactive (Tallmer, 1996) are biased perceptions often leading to failure to recognize abuse symptoms. Medical and other health care professionals often attribute bruises and fractures of elderly patients to falls. The American Medical Association (Aravanis et al., 1992) and Mount Sinai Victims Services Agency (1988) have published diagnostic and treatment guidelines on elder abuse. Ageist attitudes and biased perceptions of older adults can also result in infantilization of the elderly; consequently, decision making and choices exercised by elders may be disregarded or devalued. A loss of autonomy, one's sense of control over life, can also have negative mental health consequences. Counselors must be alert to another misconception, that depression is a consequence of aging. In fact, depression may often be the result of excessive or interactive effects of medication, physical status, loss and bereavement, lack of friendships or confidantes, or an abusive domestic environment. All of these potentially contributing factors need to be investigated.

The hypothesis that elders who are in poorer health and functionally limited in activities of daily life would be more likely to be abused was unsupported by the research of Pillemer and Finkelhor (1989) and Borden and Berlin (1990). However, there is increasing evidence that there are strong associations of abuse of elderly with developmental disabilities and those suffering from Alzheimer's disease. Ultimately, it is ageism that limits research and clinical practices with the victims and their families.

Family Violence

Therapists often fail to recognize family violence or its seriousness. In a study by Harway (1992), therapists were shown to be unprepared to intervene in areas of family violence. She reported that therapists were unable to properly assess the danger inherent in domestic violence cases and were shown to be unprepared to intervene. This is especially true when the victim is an elder (Deitch, 1993).

Using the perspective of intergenerational transmission of violence, those families who have experienced violence were believed to be more prone to that behavior than those who did not. However, Pillemer and Finkelhor's (1989) study exploring the causes for violence did not find support for intergenerational transmission of violence. Pillemer and Suitor (1989) studied the causes of violence and violent feelings among family members. Caregivers who expressed a fear of violence cited that disruptive behaviors such as wandering, outbursts, or embarrassing or assaultive behaviors were important predictors of interactional stress. Another finding was that spouses were more likely than adult children to become violent to their care recipients. Persons with lower self-esteem feared becoming violent. Living with the care recipient was positively related to violent feelings. The Pillemer and Suitor data also suggested that caregivers with more violent feelings toward their care recipients were more likely to institutionalize them.

Family conflict is often a neglected aspect of variables leading to abuse by caregivers. Of the 100 adult caregivers studied by Strassburger and Wahlhagen (1991), 40% had serious conflict with another family member. The adult child caregiver also had significantly greater burdens and poorer mental health.

Adult children who return to the parental nest, as well as those who have never left, may be functionally limited due to cognitive, emotional, or chemical impairment, or financial difficulties. They remain dependent on their elderly parents and therefore present a potentially higher risk for abusive behaviors. Family systems need to be assessed to determine whether caregiving by adult children for their elderly parent is recommended.

What emerges as an abuser profile is one in which the family member presents with a pathological history, deficient socialization, a history of mental and emotional problems, a psychological dependence on the "victim," and possibly a chemical or alcoholic addiction. Pillemer and Finkelhor (1989) reported that 20% of reported abusers had a substance addiction. The abuse of alcohol by male caregivers was a consistent finding. Deviance and dependency are more evident in the abusive family member (Simon, 1992).

Spousal Abuse

Spousal abuse is more prevalent than any other form of domestic elder abuse (New York City Department for the Aging, 1990; Pillemer & Finkelhor, 1989; Pillemer & Suitor, 1991; Sengstock, 1991). The likelihood of wives being abused by their husbands is nearly three times greater than that of husbands being mistreated by their wives (National Aging Resource Center on Elder Abuse, 1990; U.S. Department of Justice, 1991). In a study of marital homicides, Goetting (1989) reported that women had a higher rate of homicidal victimization. Those wives who do use violence may be acting in self-defense.

For some couples, the postparental years are especially devastating because of spousal abuse. Koss (1990) reported that 25–33% of married couples are affected by violence. Elderly spousal abuse may reflect a long-standing pattern of domestic violence (Pillemer & Finkelhor, 1988; Sengstock, 1991), behavior begun early in the marriage, unrecognized as abusive, and escalating with time. Nonphysical forms of abuse can be shouting, cursing, name-calling, withholding money, or withdrawing from one's partner sexually and emotionally (Deitch, 1993).

In a number of cases, elderly spousal abuse is a relatively new phenomenon. Deitch (1993) described late-onset spousal abuse (LOSA), in which the eruption of abuse may be triggered by the perpetrators' neurological and health status, financial pressures, losses, chemical dependency, medication, and the surfacing of previously unresolved couple issues. Often, a victim's dementia state and Alzheimer's disease can precipitate abuse (Pillemer & Suitor, 1991; Wolf, 1995). Abuse of power, substance addiction or alcoholism, and at least two major life setbacks are contributing factors (Ramsey-Klawsnick, 1993). LOSA can also be related to role conflict, skills deficit, retaliation, or dependency issues.

Sengstock (1991) focused on roles of sex and gender in generating elder abuse. The form of abuse most related to gender issues is spousal abuse in later life, with males more likely to engage in direct physical abuse. The condition under which the wife is the perpetrator is "reverse spousal abuse" (Sengstock, 1991) and occurs because the differential patterns of strength and power in the relationship change. Reverse spousal abuse may also be an act of retaliation. Husbands who are victims may be especially reluctant to report the abuse because of gender stereotyping.

Therapists are encouraged to examine gender stereotypes throughout the couple's life span. They need to determine whether they are gender bias-free in their work with elderly couples in domestic violence situations. To date, spousal abuse is not covered by mandatory reporting requirements. Harway's (1992) study found that 90% of therapists failed to recognize the seriousness of violence. This underscores the need for additional training of family counselors in this area, since family violence and abuse cover a wide range of interpretations (Holtzworth-Munroe & Arias, 1993).

Psychological abuse among elderly couples may remain part of an ongoing pattern or emerge because of life changes. Adult children are often called on to help their parents resolve differences. Family counselors can play a significant role in working with those adult children to help them to avoid settling the differences for their parents. Therapists can offer perspectives on the role they play in alliances, coalitions, alienation, and in fostering dependency. If the arguments between the parents are so destructive that they create tensions that extend to their children and grandchildren, it is appropriate for family members to encourage their parents to seek the services of a family therapist.

Sexual Abuse of the Older Family Member

Sexual abuse is the most hidden form of domestic elder abuse; therefore, statistics of its occurrence are inaccurate and unreliable. In general, there is a failure to recognize and report sexual abuse. Underreporting of sexual abuse among the elderly is linked to the double stigma of the incident. Stereotypes of the elderly as sexless persons and the family as loving and caring suggest that reports of

those incidents are unfounded (Sengstock, 1991). Stereotyping elderly women as sexless and unattractive, coupled with the social
and cultural taboos of incest, contribute to a lack of awareness and
investigation of suspected incidents.

Research into the nature and causes of sexual abuse has been
conducted by Sengstock (1991), Holt (1993), and Ramsey-Klawsnick
(1993). Marital rape is a common form of sexual abuse in later life.
Sengstock (1991) attributed this abuse to sexual malfunction in the
partner. Incidence of impotence, erectile strength, and frequency
of ejaculation are affected by alcoholism, hypertension, or other
physical problems and may be contributing factors to sexual abuse.
Frustration and the need to assert one's "masculinity" in the forms
of sexual power and control underlie this abusive behavior
(Sengstock, 1991).

Adult child-to-parent incest also occurs in persons 65 and older.
In an elder sexual abuse study in Great Britain, preliminary findings by Holt (1993) indicated that out of 90 cases of suspected sexual
abuse, the ratio was 6 sexually abused females to 1 male, with 85%
of all victims 75 or older. This also confirmed Ramsey-Klawsnick's
(1993) research. Aside from rape, molestation, and incest, there are
other forms of sexual abuse of older women. They may include
exhibitionism, voyeurism, displaying pornography, using victims to
produce pornography, or allowing others sexual access to victims.
Physical symptoms, body language, and verbal cues of sexual abuse
may go unnoticed (Ramsey-Klawsnik, 1993). Because rapes and other
types of sexual abuse are particularly difficult to substantiate in
this population, investigation of sexual assault of women over 65
years of age is virtually nonexistent.

The impact of domestic sexual abuse is as traumatic for the elderly as it is for younger persons. Guilt, shame, self-blame, and fear
of not being believed discourage reporting of such events. Therapists are generally unprepared to recognize the seriousness of violence and to interview appropriately in these situations.
Ramsey-Klawsnik (1993) offered guidelines for interviewing suspected victims of sexual abuse. Recovery, a slow process for the
victim, can be assured if the counselor is properly trained in treatment techniques for the sexually abused (Harway, 1992).

Issues of Culture and Ethnicity

Family counselors must be aware of the role played by a cultur-
ally diverse, pluralistic society when assessing domestic abuse.
Attitudes and belief systems of a family's cultural context influence

how the abuse is perceived, whether the victim will seek help, and to whom they will go for assistance (Hernandez, 1991; Moon & Williams, 1993). Shame, fear, mistrust, betrayal, and family values are barriers that interfere with victims seeking help. Using three different populations (African Americans, Korean Americans, and Caucasians), Moon and Williams (1993) gave subjects a series of vignettes involving elder conflict situations. Each group's pattern revealed significant differences in the way elder mistreatment was handled. In Israel, elder abuse was considered more "acceptable" if it occurred in families and "within the context of a caring relation-ship" (Neikrug & Ronen, 1993, p. 17). A conference report on elder abuse and the American Indian (National Center on Elder Abuse, 1990) indicated a need for tribal ordinances to address this hidden problem. Furthermore, the report presented a relationship between substance abuse and elder abuse.

Counselors and researchers must exercise caution in generaliz-ing their findings to fit all groups. As part of their education and training, counselors need to become familiar with studies based on each culture (Long, 1986; Stein, 1993; Wolf, 1994). A more effective classification system of abusive behavior is required to reflect di-verse populations and avoid stereotyping of minorities (Hernandez, 1991; Moon & Williams, 1993).

Implications for Counselors

With the "graying of society," increased incidence of elder abuse is anticipated (Tatara, 1991). It is important that family clinicians become knowledgeable about domestic violence and the elderly. Treatment for domestic violence of the elderly requires skill and sensitivity.

To be effective in counseling the elderly victim and family perpe-trator, therapists need to explore their own biases against older adults. Furthermore, it is essential that counselors have knowledge of developmental and clinical issues associated with the aging pro-cess. Professional education must include geropsychology, domes-tic violence, and crisis intervention for victims of sexual assault. Intervention, especially in cases of sexual abuse, requires an aware-ness of nonverbal cues and extreme sensitivity. Although domestic violence is a crime, counselors must respect the decision of the abused elder as to whether to report incidents to authorities.

Assessment is key in working with domestic violence. It must be determined which elders are at risk in their families. Family bound-aries, family conflicts, pathology, deviance of the caregiver, history of abuse, alcoholism, and drug abuse are all contributing factors that need evaluation for counselors to make appropriate assessments in elder abuse situations. Counselors must determine the type of abuse, severity of abuse, intent of the mistreatment, emotional and functional states of abused and abuser, and access to community services. Mental health practitioners also need to evaluate the level of cognitive functioning, including ordering a neuropsychological examination to determine whether the level of cognitive functioning is related to victimization.

It is strongly recommended that family counselors avail themselves of guidelines to assist them in assessment and treatment strategies in elder abuse (Aravanis et al., 1992). Breckman's staircase model provides a tool for assessment and care management planning with elder abuse victims. The victimized elderly family member is assisted through various stages of his or her traumatic situation. Guidelines are presented for detection, assessment, and intervention for patients over 60 who are abused by family members (Mount Sinai Victims Services Agency, 1988). Baladermian (1992) described how to interview the elderly parent when he or she is a victim of abuse and is also developmentally disabled.

Since domestic violence is a family issue, offending members and other family members involved with the victim require treatment. Evaluation of potential family caregivers is essential prior to decisions regarding living arrangements of elder members. In cases where a chemically or mentally impaired adult child or spouse resides in the home, additional supportive services or respite care may be appropriate precautions. Counselors need to be familiar with community resources in order to initiate referrals to programs that create informal social support groups (Breckman & Adelman, 1988). Therapists must assess each case and make referrals for at-risk clients to senior centers, religious and social clubs, and community organizations. Social support, a confidante, or peer group can reinforce the message that abuse is unacceptable and illegal.

In cases where the elderly parent is suffering from Alzheimer's disease, Wolf (1995) offered a number of techniques to prevent elder abuse by family members:

- training caregivers in behavioral management techniques to lessen the disruptive and violent behavior of the care recipient
- providing psychological/medical/social services to caregivers to treat depressive symptoms and raise self-esteem

- making respite day care and other support services available to families to reduce the number of hours of caregiving per day
- offering counseling services to assist families in placing their family member in a residential facility when caregiving tasks become overwhelming

When aging parents enter the domain of the adult child, it is essential for counselors to assess the "premorbid" family system, the nature of the adult child's marital interaction, and how the additional elderly residents will affect the family structure. Furthermore, counselors need to know which support services are available to family members to facilitate transitions (Borden & Berlin, 1990; Douglass, 1988). Frequently, the length of a caregiving stay may be 4 to 5 years longer than anticipated. The family may feel as though they have failed and become reluctant to recommend institutional placement (Kosberg, 1988). This is an opportunity for family counselors to assist families with their decision-making powers.

Conclusion

More research into elder abuse among multiethnic groups is needed. Clinicians are cautioned to avoid overestimating the degree of psychological and physical abuse among poor and minority populations. Interventions must fit the values of the group with which they work.

Family counselors advocate for their clients by providing them with a safety net. Assistance involves informing victims of their rights, making them aware of available community resources, helping them negotiate the law enforcement and legal systems, and most importantly, supporting their efforts in the decision-making process (Deitch, 1993, 1994). The process of establishing trust and respect and building a therapeutic alliance takes time. Additionally, issues of denial, shame, and resistance must be worked through. Therapist intervention must proceed in ways to strengthen and support their clients, helping them to regain power and control over their lives.

References

Anetzberger, G. (1987). *The etiology of elder abuse by adult offspring.* Springfield, IL: Charles C Thomas.

Aravanis, S. C., Adelman, R. D., Breckman, R., et al. (1992). *Diagnostic and treatment guidelines on elder abuse and neglect.* Chicago, IL: American Medical Association.

Baladermian, N. J. (1992). *Interviewing skills to use with abuse victims who have developmental disabilities.* Washington, DC: National Aging Resource Center on Elder Abuse.

Borden, W., & Berlin, S. (1990). Gender, coping and psychological well-being in responses of older adults with chronic dementia. *American Journal of Orthopsychiatry, 60,* 603–610.

Breckman, R., & Adelman, R. (1988). *Strategies for helping victims of elder mistreatment.* Newbury Park, CA: Sage.

Deitch, I. (1993, August). *Alone, assaulted and abandoned: Elder abuse and the elderly.* Paper presented at Symposium on Domestic Violence at the 101st Annual Convention, American Psychological Association, Toronto, Canada.

Deitch, I. (1994). Don't throw mamma from the train, Part II. *The Family Psychologist, 10* (1), 23–26.

Douglass, R. L. (1988). *Domestic mistreatment of the elderly: Towards prevention.* Washington, DC: Criminal Justice Services, American Association of Retired Persons.

Goetting, A. (1989). Patterns of marital homicide: A comparison of husbands and wives. *Journal of Contemporary Family Studies, 20,* 341–351.

Greenberg, J., Seltzer, M., & Greenley, J. (1993). Aging parents of adults with disabilities: The gratifications and frustrations of later-life caregiving. *The Gerontologist, 33,* 542–550.

Harway, M. (1992). Training issues in working with violent families. *Family Violence and Sexual Assault Bulletin, 8* (2), 18–20.

Hernandez, G. (1991). Not so benign neglect: Researchers ignore ethnicity in defining family caregiving burden and recommending services (Letter to the editor). *The Gerontologist, 31,* 271–272.

Holt, M. (1993). Elder sexual abuse in Britain: Preliminary findings. *Journal of Elder Abuse and Neglect, 5* (2), 63–71.

Holtzworth-Munroe, A., & Arias, I. (1993). The influence of values in the treatment of marital violence. *Family Violence and Sexual Assault Bulletin, 9* (3), 22–25.

Hudson, M. (1991). Analysis of the concepts of elder mistreatment, abuse and neglect. *Journal of Elder Abuse and Neglect, 1* (1), 5–7.

Hugh, M. D. (1991). A new myth about families of older persons. *The Gerontologist, 37,* 611–618.

Hwalek, M., Quinn, K., & Goodrich, C. (1993). *Determining effective intervention in a community based elder abuse system.* Springfield, IL: SPEC Associates.

Kosberg, J. (1988). Preventing elder abuse: Identification of high risk factors prior to placement decisions. *The Gerontologist, 28,* 43–50.

Koss, M. (1990). The women's mental health research agenda: Violence against women. *American Psychologist, 45,* 374–380.

Long, K. A. (1986). Cultural considerations in the assessment and treatment of intrafamilial abuse. *Journal of Orthopsychiatry, 56*, 131–136.

Moon, A., & Williams, O. (1993). Perception of elder abuse and help seeking patterns among African-American, Caucasian-American, and Korean-American elderly women. *The Gerontologist, 33*, 386–395.

Mount Sinai Victims Services Agency. (1988). *Elder mistreatment: Guidelines for health care professionals: Detection, assessment and intervention,* New York: New York City Elder Abuse Project.

National Aging Resource Center on Elder Abuse. (1990). *Elder abuse— Questions and answers: An information guide for professionals and concerned citizens.* Washington, DC: Author.

Neikrug, S., & Ronen, M. (1993). Elder abuse in Israel. *Journal of Elder Abuse and Neglect, 5*(3), 1–19.

New York City Department for the Aging. (1990). *Elder abuse: A profile of victims served by the New York City Department for the Aging.* New York: New York City Elder Abuse Project.

New York City Department for the Aging. (1991). *Statistics on elder abuse in New York City.* New York: New York City Department for the Aging.

Parks, S., & Pilisuk, M. (1991). Caregiver burden: Gender and psychological costs of caregiving. *American Journal of Orthopsychiatry, 61*, 501–508.

Paveza, G. J., Cohen, D., Eisendorfer, C., et al. (1992). Severe family violence and Alzheimer's disease: Prevalence and risk factors. *The Gerontologist, 32*, 493–497.

Petel, M., Casserta, M., Hutton, A., & Lund, D. (1988). Intergenerational conflict: Middle aged women caring for demented older relatives. *American Journal of Orthopsychiatry, 58*, 405–417.

Pillemer, K. (1985, Fall). Social isolation and elder abuse. *Response, 2*–4.

Pillemer, K., & Finkelhor, D. (1988). The prevalence of elder abuse: A random sample survey. *The Gerontologist, 28*, 51–57.

Pillemer, K., & Finkelhor, D. (1989). Causes of elder abuse: Caregivers' stress vs. problem relatives. *American Journal of Orthopsychiatry, 59*, 179–187.

Pillemer, K., & Suitor, J. (1989). Violence and violent feelings: What causes them among family caregivers? *Journal of Gerontology, 47*, 165–172.

Pillemer, K., & Suitor, J. (1991). Sharing residence with an adult child: A cause of psychological distress in the elderly? *American Journal of Orthopsychiatry, 61*, 144–148.

Pritchard, M. (1993). Dispelling some myths. *Journal of Elder Abuse and Neglect, 5* (2), 27–36.

Ramsey-Klawsnik, H. (1993). Interviewing elders for suspected sexual abuse: Guidelines and techniques. *Journal of Elder Abuse and Neglect, 5* (1), 5–19.

Sengstock, M. (1991). Sex and gender: Implications in cases of elder abuse. *Journal of Women and Aging, 3* (2), 25–43.

Shiferaw, B., & Mittlemark, M. (1994). The investigation and outcome of reported cases of elder abuse: The Forsyth County Aging Study. *The Gerontologist, 34*, 123–126.

Simon, M. (1992). *An exploratory study of adult protective services programs' repeat elder abuse clients.* Washington, DC: Public Policy Institute, American Association of Retired Persons.

Stein, K. (1991). *Elder abuse and neglect: A national research agenda.* Washington, DC: National Aging Resource Center on Elder Abuse.

Stein, K. (1993). *Cultural and ethnic considerations in elder abuse.* Washington, DC: National Aging Resource Center on Elder Abuse.

Steinmetz, S. (1988). Elder abuse by family caregivers: Process and intervention. *Contemporary Family Therapy, 10*, 256–271.

Strassburger, W., & Wahlhagen, M. (1991). Impact of family conflict in adult child caregiver abuse. *The Gerontologist, 37*, 770–771.

Sukosky, D. G. (1992). Elder abuse: A preliminary profile of the abusers and the abused. *Family Violence and Sexual Assault Bulletin, 8* (4), 23–26.

Tallmer, M. (1996). *Questions and answers about sex in later life.* Philadelphia: Charles Press.

Tatara, T. (1990). *Elder abuse in the United States: An issue paper.* Washington, DC: National Aging Resource Center on Elder Abuse.

Tatara, T. (1991). *Summaries of national elder abuse data: An exploratory study of state statistics.* Washington, DC: National Aging Resource Center on Elder Abuse.

Tatara, T. (1993). Understanding the nature and scope of domestic elder abuse with the use of state aggregate data: Summaries of the key findings of a national survey of State APS and aging agencies. *Journal of Elder Abuse and Neglect, 5* (4), 35–57.

Tomes, H. (1993, July). In the public interest (column). *APA Monitor,* p. 32.

Troll, L. (1993, March). *Studies of the old-old (over 85) American population and their families.* Paper presented at the 5th International Interdisciplinary Congress on Women, San Jose, Costa Rica.

U.S. Department of Justice. (1991). *Uniform crime reports, 1990,* Publication No. 282–076/ys217. Washington, DC: U.S. Government Printing Office.

Utech, H., & Garrett, R. (1992). Elder and child abuse: Conceptual and perceptual parallels. *Journal of Interpersonal Violence, 7*, 418–428.

Wolf, R. S. (1992). Victimization of the elderly: Elder abuse and neglect; social and psychological gerontology. *Review in Clinical Gerontology, 3*, 269–273.

Wolf, R. S. (1994). Elder abuse and cultural diversity considerations: A brief look at research. *National Center on Elder Abuse Exchange, 1* (2), 6–8.

Wolf, R. S. (1995). A brief look at elder abuse and Alzheimer's disease. *National Center on Elder Abuse Exchange, 2* (2), 6–12.

■ ■ ■

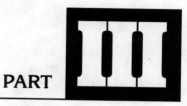

PART

AGING AND FAMILIES: TRANSITION AND TRAUMA

9

Separation and Loss in Alzheimer's Disease: Impact on the Family

Judah L. Ronch, PhD
Esther Loring Crispi, PhD

Alzheimer's disease (AD) and related disorders are fundamentally disorders of thinking and memory, but these conditions do not spare the emotional lives of either the patient or family members. AD devastates the patient's thinking, social skills, communication ability, and self-care capacity. The emotional impact on the family is profound, necessitating numerous adjustments to many losses—to loss of self, loss of a loved one, and loss of a way of life.

A major focus for intervention has been with the family. Family caregivers continue to provide the bulk of care to AD patients even when outside services are available, and they benefit from interventions that provide immediate, short-term relief from the physical stresses of caregiving and the associated emotional strain. This chapter will focus on the impact of AD on the family, including developmental considerations, counseling suggestions, and intervention strategies.

Unique Losses for the Family

AD precipitates both psychological and physical caregiving demands. The bond among family members changes significantly as the patient deteriorates. Roles evolve in unexpected directions, relationships change, and future plans must be revised.

Phases of AD

To understand the losses associated with AD, it is first necessary to define the behavioral phases of AD. Although there are no universally accepted stage descriptions of AD, and symptoms may vary, there are some common characteristics that occur at the various phases of AD. The descriptions that follow are drawn from the work of Gwyther (1985) and the Burke Rehabilitation Center (1980).

In the first phase of AD, the patient may become less socially competent, less logical, somewhat depressed, and more argumentative. Recent memory may be impaired, and the individual may get lost in familiar places, forget words, and make errors in judgment. In the second phase, the patient may become more dependent, lack logical thought, become more anxious, and have hallucinations. The individual may need care from other family members, may exhibit bizarre or embarrassing behavior, may become overly suspicious, and may sometimes become uninhibited. In the third phase, the patient may be apathetic and remote, be incontinent, have poor memory, be unable to communicate, and be unable to walk. Care at this point is likely to be of a more custodial nature.

As can be seen from the descriptions of the phases of dementia, the patient may gradually lose those characteristics that compose the "self." The personality transforms and becomes distorted, and personhood ebbs. The patient gradually loses orientation to time and place and the ability to recognize others. As this occurs, social relationships disappear. In the end, even the person's self-care becomes dependent on others.

Grief and Alzheimer's Disease

Normal grieving following death or sudden illness usually follows a pattern. Wisocki and Averill (1987, p. 132) described four stages of normal grieving. They are (a) shock—characterized by a dazed sense of unreality lasting anywhere from hours to days; (b) protest and yearning—where the loss is recognized but not entirely accepted, intense longing occurs, the loss is protested, dreaming of the lost person occurs, and the bereaved person may become preoccupied with memories of the lost person; (c) disorganization and despair—where the bereaved person may feel bitterness, apathy, withdrawal, loss of energy, despondency, and depression (appetite change, sleep disturbances, loss of libido, isolation, etc.), lasting a year or more; and (d) detachment, reorganization, and recovery—when the person begins to develop new ways of thinking about the world, establishes new relationships with a sense of purpose, and begins enjoying life again, though the pain of loss may never subside completely.

For those who have a relative with AD, the grief process may be protracted. Social support in the ongoing grieving process may not be available to caregivers because the patient may not appear ill. Additionally, the family cannot find closure and mutual disengagement. Family caregivers, especially spouses, females, and younger caregivers are at risk of experiencing a "loss of self" as roles other than caregiving are eliminated (Skaff & Pearlin, 1992).

Impact on the Family

Impact on the Spouse

Spouses of AD patients often experience negative consequences as a result of direct caregiving responsibilities, loss of companionship, and inability to continue their own personal development. The nature of how AD can affect spouses can be appreciated by how it affects normal developmental trajectories. Since spouses are typically in late adulthood themselves, this section provides examples of normal development in late adulthood, based on the work of Colarusso and Nemiroff (1981). Each area of development will be amended to include a brief description of AD's impact.

Intimacy, love, and sex. Developmental tasks in later life include the capacity to tolerate loss, death of partner and friends; the ability to form new sustaining ties with friends, children, and grandchildren; and continuation of an active sex life.

The partner of the Alzheimer's patient is often prevented from developing along these normative adulthood lines. Many of the tasks are relational and involve changes made by couples in the process of growing and adjusting to each other in new ways. The unimpaired spouse remembers the history of the relationship and also sees that future development will not occur in the way that was anticipated. The relationship cannot be redefined in a normal way once the children grow but must evolve into a caregiver–dependent relationship. The ability to care for the spouse may become the entire focus of the caregiver's life. New interests, activities, and people cannot be shared or enjoyed; friendships cannot be pursued; career challenges may be forgone.

The body. As individuals reach their seventies and beyond, the tasks typically include the ability to remain active and outgoing in the face of frequent physical infirmity, acceptance of permanent physical impairment and chronic illness, and continued exercise and care of the body.

Caregiving responsibilities often necessitate considerable energy and physical stamina. This is especially difficult in view of the fact that normal development entails some physical decline. Caregiving spouses sometimes become ill and even die as a result of increased physical requirements of caregiving. Normal development includes coming to terms with physical changes and adapting and compensating by conserving physical capacity. Caring for a demented spouse does not allow for this.

Time and death. For those in their 60s, developmental tasks related to the understanding of the passage of time and inevitability of death may include acceptance of the preciousness of time, leading to an increased interest in the quality of experience; the effect of personal vulnerability, illness, and aging on thoughts of time and death; and dealing with the effect of death of a loved one. As individuals reach their 70s and older, the tasks involve finding meaning in their lives and preparation for personal death.

Spouses of the demented perceive the passage of time as both an ally and an enemy. In the face of progressive dementia characterized as it is by continual loss, the unimpaired spouse becomes aware that there is little time to enjoy what the couple has left. Conversely, time passes too slowly for those who have come to terms with the inevitable loss of a spouse and wish for a merciful termination of the patient's suffering and deterioration. Counselors are confronted with the family's protracted grief process, time ambivalence, and the needs spouses have to integrate thoughts of the patient's death with their own.

Relationships with children. As adults reach their seventies and beyond, tasks include the continued facilitation of grown children's and grandchildren's development and the acceptance of support from middle-aged children.

Family relations with children may be severely disrupted when a parent has AD. The demented parent is unable to mature and develop normally. The spouse's normative roles as nurturer, advisor, and grandparent are compromised because of caregiving responsibilities that divert attention, monopolize energy, and use precious resources. If caregiving stress causes accelerated physical decline in the unimpaired spouse, children will be asked to undertake additional responsibilities for care.

Finances. For older adults, tasks include adaptation to retirement income and plans for money after one's own death—making a will, providing for family and community.

Play and work. As adults reach old age, the tasks include continued involvement in meaningful work and play, adjusting to retirement, adjusting to diminished capacity for mental hobbies and ability for physical play, and meaningful use of time.

Work, finances, and play are all subject to separation and loss in the lives of caregiving spouses and AD patients. Caregiving duties may result in financial loss due to the inability of the caregiver to continue on the planned career path. Money earmarked for future leisure plans eventually is depleted in the process of paying for care and supporting the family when income is interrupted, especially as insurance plans currently do not cover the oppressive costs. The spouse must cope with an insecure financial future as well as present interruption of career plans. Other insecurities revolve around the fact that eventual reentry into the work force will be difficult for elderly candidates.

Counseling Considerations

Spouses of dementia patients experience a loss of connections built up over the history of the relationship. The nondemented spouse may sense the loss of the demented spouse as a major source of support, comfort, and security. The sexual relationship may suffer as the demented spouse becomes disinterested, overinterested, catastrophically reactive, or forgets how to make love. The nondemented spouse may lose interest because of shifting roles or attempts at grief-produced disengagement.

Caregiving spouses may be unable to benefit from a marital relationship but find that they may have to abandon vocational, professional, and recreational interests for all or part of the duration of caregiving. They often complain of becoming socially isolated and may experience the need for outside social companionship, especially near the end of the patient's illness. This can lead to guilt, awkwardness, and fears of censure by others if they try to reengage socially while the patient is still alive.

The process of counseling can be assisted by an understanding that development continues throughout the life span. The caregiving spouse of an AD patient may find personal development significantly affected by day-to-day struggles. Continuous loss and lack of normal grieving opportunities compounded by interrupted development can produce emotional difficulties for the nondemented spouse. Counseling can provide both short- and long-term benefits by considering resumption of developmental tasks as an intervention goal along with the work of coping with the illness and its effects. Active listening and feedback that puts caregiver burden and frustration within this context can help to place problems in perspective and provide a systematic approach to goal clarification.

A particularly difficult area for caregivers to consider is the transfer of responsibility of some aspect of the patient's care to another caregiver or agency. Clinicians may find that this occurs when the burden of caregiving exceeds the caregiver's physical, emotional, or financial resources. Guilt feelings, which are common among caregivers (Brody, 1988; Cohler, Groves, Borden, & Lazarus, 1989), may increase when there is a necessity to institutionalize the AD spouse. Counselors often must illuminate "covert contracts" among family members that are at the root of such guilt.

Children of the Patient

Children of AD patients, many of whom are in middle adulthood, face many of the same issues related to grieving that spouses do, such as stress related to caregiving and grief related to loss of the parent's affection and companionship. Additionally, they may also experience strains related to role conflicts. Because most adults in midlife are married with grown children, caring for an AD parent may prevent the midlife adult from spending time with his or her own family.

Since children will likely experience losses associated with developmental growth, it is also valuable to look at normative adult development in midlife in order to see the potential impact of AD on adult children. Crispi and Fisher (1994) have provided some of the major categories of adult development in midlife that can be affected by caregiving responsibilities described in this section.

Career goals. Many adults in their 40s and 50s are satisfied with their careers, both financially and in terms of fulfillment and prestige. Others may seek to start new careers because of changes in family structure, interests, and a realistic assessment of the number of years of productive work remaining for them. Additionally, some may feel threatened by younger coworkers who may be more physically fit or technologically advanced. Individuals who have spent early adulthood raising children full-time may now be reentering the work force, or entering for the first time.

Leisure time. Midlife adults may find that they are able to pursue leisure time activities that had previously been unattainable due to time restrictions and financial considerations. These activities may be very fulfilling and a way of expressing oneself.

Sexuality and adjustment to physical change. Adults in middle age experience a gradual decline in physical ability including, for some, sexual capability. For others, the decline may be more psychological in nature. Adjustment to aging and changes in sexual functioning are aided by mutual communication and understanding of these issues with the sexual partner.

Parenting. The parenting process changes as children grow and move away. The spouses are left alone to focus on being a couple again and to learn how to live with each other, as well as how to deal with adult children. Some families find that adult children remain in the home and additional adjustments need to be made.

Delayed childbearing. Some adults do not become parents until in their 40s, and have children who are in elementary and high school when they are in their 50s. For many of these late childbearing adults, responsibilities for child-rearing occur simultaneously with growing career responsibilities.

Aging parents. For some midlife adults, aging parents become dependent on them at the time in their lives when career goals are prominent, when children are growing or have left home, and when they anticipate enjoying leisure time and other postponed life fulfillments.

Counseling Considerations

Burdens of caring for an elderly parent may be physical, psychological, and financial. Caregiving experiences vary widely and depend on the individuals involved, their situations, the social supports received, and the nature and manifestation of the parent's illness or dependency needs.

Development in midlife can be viewed as a time of both challenge and adjustment to change. Successful resolution of issues related to career, leisure, sexual and physical change, parenting, childbearing, and parent care depend in large part on personal abilities and resources. The process can be immeasurably more difficult for the individual who has to deal with a parent who has AD. Adult children may be severely affected by a parent with AD whether or not they reside in the same household. The emotional impact of observing a parent progressively deteriorate mentally produces distress for the adult child and puts a strain on their spouse and children.

The parent–child relationship may become developmentally static yet seemingly frantic at times when the parent has AD. The child feels increasing pressure to provide care and to adjust to an environment of crisis and need. Counselors will find that the child may experience marital and family stress, reduced job performance, anxiety, depression, and withdrawal of interest from the spouse, children, and the community. Counselors will have to help the adult child cope with feelings and conflicts regarding the demented parent, personal life circumstances, and stressors related to development.

Children and Adolescents

For the most part, children and adolescents who seek counseling will be grandchildren of the AD patient, although there are some for whom the patient is a parent. Developmental issues discussed in this section apply equally well regardless of the child's relationship to the AD patient.

Counselors often have to assist children in understanding the losses they are experiencing when a relative has dementia. Young children may become frightened, confused, and regressed in reaction to a dementing relative. Poor school performance and behavioral difficulties such as hostility, uncooperativeness, or withdrawal from others may be evidenced. Psychosocial development may be affected because normal family roles change. Identity formation and development of positive self-esteem may be adversely affected. The child may also suffer from lack of affection and guidance from the parent who spends a major amount of time as a caregiver to the AD relative. This may lead to anger, frustration, sadness, and guilt reactions in the child that may require counseling.

Children of all ages may struggle over the seemingly contradictory experiences of having an AD relative physically present but emotionally and psychologically fading away. The patient may display markedly different behavior when dementing, yelling without reason, behaving in a bizarre way, or embarrassing the child in public. Children may fear what the relative has become and often also fear that it will happen to them or their parents. The once-secure life of the child is transformed into one in which individuals are vulnerable to unpredictable, drastic, negative changes.

Adolescents have many of the same experiences related to dementia that younger children do, but they may react differently.

Adolescents are typically concerned with the developmental issues of overcoming identity confusion and establishing a stable personal identity. This process involves a gradual restoration of trust in one's body that has been shaken by puberty, as well as a gradual shift to the peer group for socialization. Children of this age group need time and the space to experiment with various values and roles in the identity formation process. When confronted with a relative with AD, adolescents may feel that the human body is not necessarily to be trusted. Additionally, they may be diverted from identity exploration to a family environment where everyone's help is needed. Adolescents may need to supplement family income, assist the parental caregiver, and perform other household duties. Family duties may prevent the adolescent from spending time with the peer group and may force the adolescent to miss social, athletic, vocational, and community activities that typically promote psychosocial development and identity formation. Conflict can ensue when the adolescent experiences the struggle between pressures to help with caregiving at home and the desire to be free to pursue normal adolescent activities outside the home.

Children and adolescents sometimes find that the grandparent with AD moves into their home permanently. Many children react positively and form good relationships with the grandparent. Some may adjust graciously if they have to sacrifice their room, free time, or customary activities for their grandparent, yet others may resent the changes and react with something akin to sibling rivalry.

Counselors should assess the impact on the child within the context of the three-generational family system. Valuable information can include the age of the child, the relationship with the parents and grandparents, proximity to the grandparent with AD, and frequency of visits. Children's feelings should be considered in family counseling sessions regarding these issues. Educational approaches that give the child information about AD on a developmentally appropriate age level can help them understand behavioral changes in the grandparent. Guthrie (1986) and Van Ornum and Mordock (1994) have provided insights for counselors who are helping children cope with sharing a home with a demented grandparent.

The Counseling Process

Counselors approach the process of family intervention in numerous ways. However, there are some commonalities. All approaches involve assessment procedures and intervention strategies, and most counselors will need to deal with the grieving process with both adults and children. The following discussion highlights some elements of each part of the counseling process that are especially effective in dealing with families of AD patients, including special considerations in counseling children.

Assessment

Information regarding family history and current family functioning is useful to the family counselor, whether the client is a single family member, a marital pair, siblings, or members of multiple generations. Developmental milestones such as births, deaths, marriages, retirements, graduations, and job changes provide valuable data on family evolution. Counselors can work with family members to define the dynamics of their particular family system, including relationships within the nuclear and extended family, emotional ties, and social or community networks. With this knowledge, the counselor can teach the family how the systems and subsystems operate and help the family to resolve communication conflicts and emotional difficulties. This knowledge of family relationships and support networks helps the counselor put the patient and client in context within the dynamic family system and suggests points for intervention strategies. Counselors are referred to Nichols (1984) for a more complete description of extended family therapy.

Counselors will find it helpful to determine from caregivers the reasons for which they assumed the caregiving role. Some possible reasons could include being chosen by the family, volunteering, demonstrating devotion or providing an extension to the marital bond, martyrdom, or becoming a caregiver because no one else could do it. Exploration of these issues will provide a way for the caregiver to express feelings regarding the caregiving role.

Other family members will each play a unique part in the dynamics of the caregiving system. Some roles may be complementary and facilitative, while others may obstruct the caregiving process. The nature of these relationships, and how the individuals interact with each other as well as with the patient, should be assessed by the counselor and may become a focus of treatment.

In the initial interview, the counselor should work with the clients to focus on the problem areas that they wish to solve. Counseling should be a partnership in which counselor and clients work together to solve the difficulties directly related to dementia. The counselor needs to differentiate problems that are new, continuing, or reactivated (Steinman, 1979). Appropriate goals based on newer stressors directly related to dementia are presumably more amenable to change, and resolving these problems may provide emotional relief earlier than would attempts to resolve long-standing family difficulties.

A realistic appraisal of the family's ability and willingness to assume caregiving responsibilities and cope with the stressors of dementia can be developed (Cohen, 1983). Assessment may include the following: degree of organization or disorganization of the family system; family members' understanding of and ability to understand medical and psychological problems; level of dysfunction and residual capacities of the patient; interpersonal disruption of the family caused by dementia; cooperation within the family; dynamics of subsystems within the family to each other and the patient; presence of psychopathology within the family; presence of major physical illness, acute or chronic, within the family; current status of marital relations within the family; nature of family communications systems—the way emotions are expressed, role designations, family myths, secrets, images; traumatic events, past and present, within the family; and recent or recurrent crises in the life of any family member.

Each family member will have a unique pattern of stressors and helpful components that contribute to the overall family system. Taken together, the counselor can assess the capacity and willingness of the family to work together and assume the care of the patient with AD. Once this is done, family goals can be established in a realistic way with regard to expectations, need for community support from service providers, and feelings about assistance from outside agencies. The family can then work with the counselor to explore options for care including combinations of home care and community assistance, or in some cases, institutionalization. The counselor should also be sensitive to the possibility of abusive family situations, which may occur in the stressed environment of the family dealing with an elder with AD (Stilwell, 1990).

Counseling Interventions

Both primary prevention and intervention strategies can assist family caregivers. Caregiver burden can be prevented or reduced in a number of ways, as members share practical tips, personal experiences, and invaluable emotional support with each other. Problem-solving strategies can help caregivers deal with stressors, especially behavioral disruptions by the patient. They may also be beneficial as a general model in helping the family solve caregiving problems and exploring options. The steps include identifying problem behaviors (type and frequency), generating solutions, selecting the most appropriate solution, cognitive rehearsal of the solution to identify problems, encouragement to carry out the plan, and outcome evaluation (Zarit, 1987). Bibliotherapy sources (Cohen & Eisdorfer, 1986; Mace & Rabins, 1991; Ronch, 1991) should be recommended to help families with practical intervention ideas. Referral to an Alzheimer's support group run by local chapters of the Alzheimer's Association can be of significant benefit as group members share advice and experiences and lend emotional support and validation.

Grief Counseling

Counselors may need to assist with numerous grief reactions by family members as dementia progresses. Counselors should strive to help the family learn to grieve without feeling guilt at each point of loss. The process of gradual separation from the patient may evoke strong, often inexpressible, emotions in various family members. When expressed, the feelings may include rage, panic, and hate for the disease or the patient.

Adult children of AD patients may need assistance in dealing with conflictual emotions regarding the deterioration and death of the parent. For example, they may have to deal with the no-win situation in which medical treatment could extend the parent's life without altering the course of cognitive deterioration. Counselors can also help clients explore ambivalent feelings about their parents, fears about becoming dementia victims themselves, impending orphanhood, and their own mortality. Mullen (1992) provided an analysis of the relationship between AD caregiving and bereavement adaptation that may help counselors to understand caregiver responses to the deterioration and death of an AD relative. Responses include the coexistence of feelings of overload, depression, guilt, and mastery (personal control) among caregivers attempting to adapt to the death of an AD relative.

The adult child who witnesses the deterioration and death of a parent must also confront personal aging and mortality issues. Counselors may find that the adult child feels disturbed by thinking of personal issues at a time when the parent is so ill. Counseling can help adult children accept their feelings without guilt and self-deprecation.

Adults may find it difficult to express themselves to outsiders, including counselors, especially when counseling shifts from concrete issues to personal feelings. Family members may find that the counseling process is in direct conflict with perceived obligations to keep family secrets. They may want to present an acceptable public persona in counseling, rather than risk exposure of their negative feelings about other family members. Clients will benefit from reassurance that angry feelings about a relative with dementia are normal and can coexist with feelings of love.

Adult children often feel that they should be able to repay the demented parent in the identical manner that they were cared for as children. It is unrealistic to expect this, especially when a parent has dementia. Even if they received conditional love as children, they need to know that payback in terms of role reversal is not possible. Counselors can guide adult children to other methods of reciprocating in spirit, with fairness and justice, and show them that continued attempts at impossible goals will only lead to frustration.

Counseling Children

Children may demonstrate sensitivity, insight, and honesty, which facilitate the counseling process. Adolescents are especially inclined to be sensitive and shy but also may tend to be aggressive in counseling because of their insecurities and fear of looking foolish to others (Van Ornum & Mordock, 1994). Children of all ages can cope with the illness better if other family members relate to them openly on a level they can understand. Family counseling provides a forum for the child to share experiences, ask questions, and observe other family members dealing with the issues. The child can also discover productive, even unique, ways to assist in caregiving.

Children's issues may differ from other family members, because they view the world from the perspective of their developmental level. They may not understand the larger implications of a grandparent who is disoriented to time or who wanders passively, but they may react to the concrete behavior. Adolescents may find counseling helpful despite initial misgivings. It can help the youngster express feelings of frustration, fears, sadness, and anger. Counselors can encourage adolescents to ask questions about AD and to educate themselves on the topic. It is not unusual for adolescents to harbor strong conflictual feelings about parents, the family member with AD, and others within the family system. Some time alone with the counselor can be beneficial in providing the adolescent a way to express these feelings in privacy.

Conclusion

AD is a devastating illness causing extreme difficulties for families and bringing numerous family members to counseling. The burdens and presenting complaints will tend to differ for various family members depending on their individual temperament, relationship to the AD patient, position within the family, personal developmental level, and existing support networks both within the family and with social or community sources.

The counselor who provides services for families of AD patients is particularly challenged to develop assessment techniques and intervention strategies that address the unique needs of individual family members. Knowledge of the pattern of losses and difficulties associated with grieving will assist the counselor in understanding the uniqueness of their grief. Understanding normal development at each life stage (e.g., Crispi & Fisher, 1994; Levinson, 1986) can assist the counselor in formulating strategies to help family members set developmental goals to promote individual growth.

References

Brody, E. M. (1988). The long haul: A family odyssey. In L. F. Jarvik & C. H. Winograd (Eds.), *Treatments for the Alzheimer patient* (pp. 107–122). New York: Springer.

Burke Rehabilitation Center. (1980). *Managing the person with intellectual loss at home*. White Plains, NY: Author.

Cohen, D. (1983). Management of stress in families caring for relatives with Alzheimer's disease and related disorders. In G. Landsberg (Ed.), *Preventing mental health problems in the elderly: Directions and strategies* (pp. 74–83). Nutley, NJ: Huffman Laroche.

Cohen, D., & Eisdorfer, C. (1986). *The loss of self: A family resource for the care of Alzheimer's disease and related disorders*. New York: Plume Publishing.

Cohler, B. J., Groves, L., Borden, W., & Lazarus, L. (1989). Caring for family members with Alzheimer's disease. In E. Light & B. D. Lebowitz (Eds.), *Alzheimer's disease treatment and family stress: Directions for research* (pp. 50–105). Rockville, MD: U.S. Department of Health and Human Services.

Colarusso, C., & Nemiroff, R. (1981). *Adult development*. New York: Plenum.

Crispi, E. L., & Fisher, C. B. (1994). Development in adulthood. In J. L. Ronch, W. Van Ornum, & N. C. Stilwell (Eds.), *The counseling sourcebook* (pp. 343–357). New York: Crossroad/Continuum.

Guthrie, D. (1986). *Grandpa doesn't know me*. New York: Human Sciences Press.

Gwyther, L. (1985). *Care of Alzheimer's patients: A manual for nursing home staff*. Washington, DC: The American Health Care Association and the Alzheimer's Disease and Related Disorders Association.

Levinson, D. J. (1986). A conception of adult development. *American Psychologist, 41*, 3–13.

Mace, N., & Rabins, P. (1991). *The thirty-six hour day* (Rev. ed). Baltimore: Johns Hopkins University Press.

Mullen, J. T. (1992). The bereaved caregiver: A prospective study of changes in well-being. *The Gerontologist, 32*, 673–683.

Nichols, M. (1984). Extended family systems therapy. In M. Nichols (Ed.), *Family therapy: Concepts and methods* (pp. 345–392). New York: Gardner Press.

Ronch, J. L. (1991). *Alzheimer's disease: A practical guide for families and other caregivers*. New York: Crossroad/Continuum.

Skaff, M. M., & Pearlin, L. I. (1992). Caregiving: Role engulfment and the loss of self. *The Gerontologist, 32*, 656–664.

Steinman, L. (1979). Reactivated conflicts with aging parents. In P. Ragen (Ed.), *Aging parents* (pp. 126–143). Los Angeles: University of Southern California Press.

Stilwell, N. C. (1990). *Predictive classification of abused and non-abused elders: Elder characteristics, abuser characteristics and life satisfaction*. Unpublished doctoral dissertation, Hofstra University, Hempstead, NY.

Van Ornum, W., & Mordock, J. (1994). Counseling adolescents. In J. L. Ronch, W. Van Ornum, & N. C. Stilwell (Eds.), *The counseling sourcebook* (pp. 286–297). New York: Crossroad/Continuum.

Wisocki, P., & Averill, J. (1987). The challenge of bereavement. In L. Cartensen & B. Edelstein (Eds.), *Handbook of clinical gerontology* (pp. 312–321). New York: Pergamon.

Zarit, S. (1987). The burden of caregivers. In A. Kalicki (Ed.), *Confronting Alzheimer's disease* (pp. 109–119). Owings Mills, MD: National Health Publishing.

■ ■ ■

10

Couple Therapy With the Intact Caregiver and the Frail Cared-For: A Case Study

Marcella Bakur Weiner, EdD, PhD

C ognitive disorders are frequent concerns for therapists working with the elderly (Sadavoy, Lazarus, & Jarvik, 1992). This
type of impairment can be caused by at least 70 known ailments,
including primary brain diseases as well as diseases of other organ
systems causing secondary brain dysfunction. Called dementia, this
is a deterioration in intellectual performance that always involves
memory loss, a loss of problem-solving ability, and loss of other
aspects of abstract thinking.

Alzheimer's disease (AD) is the most common form of dementia.
Approximately 15% of the U.S. population aged 65 and over, or 4.4
million persons, are estimated to suffer from senile dementia. The
symptoms of AD include gradual declines in memory, learning, attention, and judgment; disorientation in time and space; word-find-
ing and communication difficulties; and changes in personality
(Aronson, 1988). To compound this problem is the recognized fact
that, for much of the time, there appears to be little correlation
between behavior and the extent of lesions of the brain, despite
diagnostic workups such as neuroimaging techniques, mental status testing, and clinical evaluation (Weiner, Teresi, & Streich, 1983).

Despite views to the contrary, the family is still the most important social group for older people, and most critically, families do not usually abandon their elder members (Doty, 1986; Ferraro, 1990; Horowitz, 1985; Stone, Cafferata, & Sangi, 1987; Weiner, Teresi, & Streich, 1983). Where physical or mental frailty exists in a family member and where there is a living spouse, he or she is first in line as caretaker, followed by sons and daughters, siblings, and trailed by other relatives and friends (Weiner, Teresi, & Streich, 1983).

It was this that manifested itself in the therapy with Amy and Frank, a longtime married elderly couple who were, for the very first time in their lives, in a desperate situation.

Amy and Frank: A Case Study

When I received the "cry for help," it was from the spouse, Amy's husband. Frank's voice was unsteady on the phone, but desperation could be sensed as he explained that his daughter, living in California, and his son, living in Canada, who "did come to New York to see their parents every now and then," had suggested that he see a therapist. An appointment was arranged.

Amy, 76, and Frank, 78, were a striking-looking couple, the kind about whom one thinks, "They must have been stunning in their earlier years." Frank was tall and slim, with cropped gray hair and a pensive, if somewhat sad, look to his face. He appeared agile and in full control, qualities that would turn out to be most crucial to his sense of self. Amy was quite beautiful, with neatly cut white hair, the short bangs framing her face, easily accentuating her clear gray eyes. Attractively dressed, she clutched her small purse to herself, appearing unwilling to release it any time, as though afraid she would not know where she had placed it—an observation that turned out to be most valid.

The Problem: A Two-Sided View

Folk wisdom has it that people generally have two reasons for doing anything: the reason that sounds good and the real reason. Of all the different techniques of therapy, probably the most powerful is encouraging the hidden agenda to emerge. But first came Frank and Amy's "sounds good" reason. Said Frank: "I came here because my children suggested it (pause) and I guess we need some help. Amy is having difficulty with memory and I want very much to help her (long pause) but I'm not sure what to do." At that point he stopped and looked helplessly at Amy. She replied with a shrug of her shoulders, clutched her pocketbook even more tightly in her rolled-up fist, and said quickly: "I'm here because Frank wants me to be here. I don't know why I'm here. I really am quite all right. You seem like a nice woman, but I don't think I need anyone." The rest of that session was spent obtaining background information. I discovered that theirs had been a long-term marriage and that their son and daughter, both divorced, had provided them with grandchildren of whom they were very fond. Though visits by any of them were rare, there had been more frequent phone calls of late. When visits did occur, two or three times a year, they were lovingly received. Disappointments over infrequency were never expressed. Similarly, most of their adult friends had ceased visiting them and phone calls were also on a decline. Both Amy and Frank had been teachers for many years until retirement; he had taught mathematics to high school students and she was an elementary school teacher. Both had fully enjoyed their work.

A short time into therapy, the "real reason" for coming into treatment emerged, despite the fact that Amy continued to deny that there was any necessity for doing so. Reluctantly, Frank explained that he felt imprisoned in a jail not of his making. He stated that Amy's demands for his constant attention were "making my life unbearable as though there were no openings in this prison, not even time for short recreational periods which even prisoners are allowed." Amy, in turn, bitterly contested this with: "He goes out all the time, leaving me all alone, not caring about me, and the only reason he is here is because he wants to get rid of me." This ended with an explosive: "Go! Who cares?"

The Heart of the Problem

After several sessions it became apparent that Amy represented many women in treatment who had not been adequately represented in the gerontological literature, that is, her presentation of self did not reflect her real self (Weiner, Brok, & Snadowsky, 1987). Socially, she was most adept and sophisticated. It was evident that her many years of expertise in this area had not worn off. Any attempt to delve into details that she obviously could not remember were counteracted with a smile and an offhand dismissal: "Well, my dear, you would know the answer to that better than I." It was apparent very early on that her memory was, indeed, most deficient. Deep impairments of short- and long-term memory, abstract thinking, and judgment deeply cut into the fabric of her everyday life.

After a few treatment sessions, with the approval of the couple, the family physician and I were in touch, along with other professionals who had seen Amy and Frank. I was thus aware of all the diagnostic procedures Amy had been subjected to along with the results. It became obvious that, once again, neurological examinations did not reflect the extent of her disturbed behavior patterns. For example, Amy could never find her way to the office bathroom. She would stroll along the short corridor leading from the office to that room with seeming determination that this, indeed, was the way. In this search, each closet was opened, as was the front door, until she found the bathroom, most often assisted by Frank and me. At one time she wandered outdoors until both Frank and I, at first unaware of her wandering but sensing that something was wrong, jumped up to see where she was. We caught her descending the few steps leading to the street and brought her back upstairs. In discussion, it became apparent that Frank's attempts to bring someone into the house to relieve him, if only for a few hours, were met by Amy's cries of abandonment that he just did not love her and fury at his "having another woman."

An Empathic Approach

Despite the fact that her memory impairment was quite severe, we focused, using a self psychology approach (White & Weiner, 1986), on the empathic stance. In this approach, empathy is not only a mode of gathering data through introspection into the needs of another but also can create an emotional bond between people. Amy's rages against Frank, expressed as "Let him just go—get out of my life—who cares— I don't need him—he just pretends he loves me, I know better," were received in therapy with an understanding of Amy's recent deep narcissistic deprivations, that unforgiving fury that arises when the control over the mirroring selfobject is lost.

Amy, suffering her multitudes of losses, was now most painfully deprived of that continuing need for applause, which, like oxygen, is essential not only in childhood and early adulthood but all through life. It was this wish to shine and be recognized, which Amy had experienced throughout her life through her beauty, charm, brightness, and social agility, that was no longer accessible. Appreciative responses from others, reliable and continuous, were now at a standstill. The audience had disappeared and no reason was given.

I felt I had to walk a sensitive line between nurturing Amy's shattered self-esteem and offering pat, unreal soothings of the "all will be well" nature. As is obvious in couple therapy, there were two persons seeking help, both deserving of equal attention, both in need of care and empathy.

In some ways, Amy was easier to manage and respond to than Frank. Vociferous in her response, she was definitive in her approach to life. There was no middle road, a thing either was or wasn't. Although this made for some difficulty, her views were never muddled or ambivalent. The line to her and away from her was direct. So was her reaction to me. Each emotion took its place. Love, resentment, jealousy, dependence, terror, sadness, each one taking its turn, surged through into the open air unrestrained and uncontaminated by an examining brain. Though it was sometimes difficult, I attempted to stay even, nurturing, empathic, and calm. I felt that Amy had enough tumult going on inside her without adding to it. Where confrontation may sometimes be used with younger patients as a means of shocking them into reality, this was not attempted with Amy. It was felt that this would have little result due to her inability to focus or retain anything for more than a minute and would be most harmful to her state of being.

Amy easily elicited soothing responses to her confusion and anger from me: "It must be terrifying to you when, as you just said, you sometimes cannot remember your son's name." When this was said, Amy usually responded with alertness and in-depth sadness, congruent with her established condition. She was, almost always, "an easy read." Frank was another matter. Because therapists working with aging patients must be mindful not to be inadvertently patronizing to them (Muslin, 1992) in the form of being overly solicitous, particularly with persons who have physical problems or lapses in their cognitive skills, I was mindful of my manner with Amy and also aware of any attitude that might arise in the treatment of Frank.

Where Amy's softness, belying her expressed toughness/vulnerability and continuous fragmentation-of-self, was manifest, Frank was a martyred stoic, expressing his need to "escape jail" on the one hand and vehemently rejecting all plans for avenues of escape on the other. Totally rejecting the fact that Amy's incapacitation was real and, more important, not very amenable to modifications of behavior or personality change, he responded to all of her accusations and queries as to his whereabouts, his uncaring attitude toward her, and his "disappearances" with annoyed, reality-based appeals. When she said, "You were gone all day yesterday," he would respond with a defended, "No, I wasn't. I was only gone when I went out to shop at 2:00 and then I was back by 3:00." To her look of confused disbelief, he would add, "I stayed in the rest of the time. I was with you so why do you say these things? I don't understand you." He would then look to me with a wounded expression, saying "I don't know why she says these things. They just aren't so."

After a short time in treatment, I asked to see Frank alone. It became apparent that he was paralyzed with guilt, confusion, and the conflicting feelings of wanting to totally leave her (i.e., divorce) along with feeling the pressure to stay with her every moment, to the neglect of his own self. It was explained to him that Amy's condition would most likely not improve, and that, as all other professionals had suggested, he would have to consider her in any plans as well as considering his own needs. Although his marriage had been fairly good, her failings at this point of life, when he was retired and looking forward to the pleasures of leisure time and indulging in his favorite pastime, reading by himself without any interruptions, proved to render him feeling hopeless and helpless.

Offering Solutions

During these individual sessions, we concentrated on ways in which Frank could help Amy. I suggested that he leave notes clearly hung up in different parts of the house as to the time of his leaving and returning along with setting clocks indicating this. I further explained to him that, to the memory-impaired person, out of sight is out of mind (Powell, 1993). Additionally, I suggested ways in which Frank could physically and emotionally soothe Amy, as she expressed her need for him. During couple therapy, he said he would be willing to try. In private sessions, Frank stated that it would be hard for him to satisfy Amy's physical demands on him such as sexual performance, saying that he "felt no passion for her." I accepted this, then asked him which physical gestures (e.g., holding hands, hugging her, and lying next to her) would be pleasing to Amy while also offering him some pleasure. He said that he would try being physically closer to her and that this would be "O.K." with him. I responded to this with warmth and encouragement, emphasizing that he was not to bypass his own sense-of-self in this giving.

We then attempted to focus on helping him in his verbal exchanges with Amy. I suggested that he not engage in verbal battle with her but try to understand her frightening disorientation due to her continuous inner fragmentation. He could respond with clear, direct, and soothing statements: "I don't want to leave you alone. I know that scares you and I understand that. We'll work something out where I will be with you. When I do have to go out, someone else will be here until I get back. You will be taken care of." Frank agreed that this approach could be more effective and that he would try it.

As Frank's own fears became crystallized and he established rapport and trust in the therapeutic alliance, the armor softened, aided by my attention to the newly focused theme of "But what about me?" To this, I replied, "Yes. What about you? What can we do to give you some joy in life along with satisfying your understandable responsibility to provide good care for your wife?" This was first done in the individual sessions with Frank since, when Amy was with him and he spent much time talking about himself, she would sob, "I don't remember any of this," so upsetting Frank that he could not go on. When she was not sobbing and Frank was speaking, she either clutched her purse, stared vacantly into space, or left the room, again to search for the bathroom, leaving us concerned about her whereabouts. In contrast, the individual sessions, held between couple sessions, seemed to relax Frank. He could then pay attention to just himself, a welcome relief, he said, from his caregiver role.

His background revealed that he had always been a fairly stoic man. When parents or siblings became ill, he covered his upset by removing himself emotionally and physically from the scene. Healthy himself, he did not have much familiarity with the world of frailties. A loner, he was close to the "lifestyle-isolate" seen by many professionals working with the elderly, a person who chooses to be alone rather than with others, in contrast to the aging person who becomes isolated through deaths of others and not by choice (Weiner, Brok, & Snadowsky, 1987). Frank began to make conscious choices. These were to read by himself, do some painting and drawing, and spend much "quiet time." This had been easily permitted in their earlier years. Amy, always gregarious, socially skilled, fun to be with, and much sought after by others, had been an active, independent woman before her disability occurred, willing to allow Frank to be the same. Frank emphasized that the clutching, clinging behavior was new in their relationship. I gradually knew how disquieting and frightening this must be to him, a man who revelled in his own independence, treasuring his aloneness and quiet time as necessary parts of himself.

Sameness and Change

The task now appeared to be one that occurs frequently in working with the elderly: how to encourage and solidify the two themes necessary for continuing and enjoying one's life at a later age. These themes are those of continuity-of-self (sameness) and simultaneous change. That is, one remains true to a core self or a definitive way of being, a continuity, while also being involved in an ongoing dynamic process, the change. This is in contradistinction to the formerly held view that the ultimate stages of development are reached in childhood. This "new" adult is a "dynamic, constantly changing and developing organism—potentially until the time of death" (Nemiroff & Colarusso, 1994, p. 100).

I used this approach to develop a new schema for Frank's daily life, while simultaneously encouraging him not to violate the essence of who he was. To begin with, I strongly advocated his getting some help. This initially consisted of telling his son and daughter and their grown grandchildren how difficult the situation actually was, asking them to visit more frequently when possible, while also being able to accept their response of a negative or positive nature. Since Amy seemed very attached to her son, it was suggested that Frank make this known to him. The son's recent divorce made Frank feel, as is familiar to many parents, that "he did not want to burden his son further." He finally came to see that his son could make a choice and that one possibility might be more frequent visits and phone calls. Frank was more comfortable with his daughter, and a similar suggestion was made to him about involving her in the situation. As happens frequently, when openly approached on these issues, both the children and grandchildren were pleased to become aware of the true facts and responded in a positive way. This process involved Frank's doing something about a situation instead of remaining fixed, stoically accepting, and feeling utterly hopeless. While this necessitated changing some behaviors and attitudes, it allowed him to pursue the very things he so treasured, maintaining his own, longtime-developed sense of who he was and his much-needed continuity.

Most urgently suggested was the need for some paid-for outside help. A part-time companion-caretaker was found, and Frank was offered ways in which he could slowly, gracefully and with care, wean himself away from being with Amy every moment of the day and evening. Slowly, he again began painting and drawing in his private studio room. Whereas Amy had previously burst in, pleading with him to be with her, he could now do this when she went on daily outings with her newly found caregiver. Later in treatment he brought in some paintings and drawings to show me and, at one time, offered me one that, he stated, was "done just for you as a way of showing my appreciation." It was accepted with gratitude.

For Amy, her former style of gregariousness was somewhat restored when, with outside help, she could again visit museums, sip tea at an outdoor café, and see the world beyond her home. With her companion she could also do some visiting and have others visit her. The presence of a caring person who would tend to Amy's needs at any given moment released visitors from feeling the pressure of Amy's disability. Instead, they could experience the pleasure of her outgoing, love-of-life-self and do this within a reasonable time frame. Prior to this, Frank would do some errands or just go for a walk when visitors appeared, making them feel "tied in" until he returned; they would then rush to escape, taking their guilt and conflicting emotions along with them. Some would never return.

"Changes" for Amy would come about mostly from a change of situation. Her inner state would, most probably, continue to fragment or, optimally, stabilize. Despite this, her world could change since she now received more genuine care from Frank and also had the opportunity to engage in activities most consonant with her intrinsic self. Her family, made aware of the real nature of the situation, could offer more loving support, thus upholding her fragile, vulnerable self. Her granddaughter, for example, a favorite of Amy's and now in her 20s, even offered to care for Amy on extended visits. This was most gratefully and enthusiastically accepted by both grandparents.

Guidelines for Therapists

When working with the elderly, therapists will often see family members who suffer from a disability. Whether in couple or family therapy, the practitioner must be careful about targeting the "identified patient" (IP) as the only one needing focused attention. This is more difficult than when working with younger, more able persons where one member's needs do not seem so acute. Still, the principle remains the same; it is the family (i.e., couple, spouse, children, or others) that needs to be addressed as being an essential part of the IP's syndrome. The needs, feelings, fears, hopes, and hurts of family members must be attended to with the same care and loving support as those of the the patient. In short, everyone must be put into the picture.

For help to be maximized, the therapist needs to be aware of some of the services available to the elderly and, where deemed appropriate, take some direct action. Making phone calls, contacting other professional agencies and asking other family members to partake in some therapy sessions should not be ruled out. This is done after receiving the consent of the patients in treatment. Direct assistance is also possible and often advisable. In Amy's case, for example, I helped her walk to the bathroom and assisted her in finding the light. I later would help her search for the book or newspaper she may have brought to the session and which Amy said "had just disappeared."

Although I find that understanding the inner workings of the person's world from a self psychology perspective is most helpful, I do not focus on the past with the elderly or always express my insights. Rather, I often contain them within myself while choosing the most-needed therapeutic path to take. Focusing on the here-and-now, I am appreciative of the fact that "life stories" can be a useful tool and are considered one way of doing effective psychotherapy with the elderly (Viney, 1993). However, in cases such as Amy and Frank's, it may have limited value during conjoint couple therapy sessions. In this case, when Frank would spend much time on stories related to background, Amy would sob and ask, "When did this all happen?" causing Frank to go pale and freeze. It was too much for Amy to handle. Conversely, during individual sessions with Frank, his life stories were gathered and appreciated, providing insights into his past, which were most helpful, along with some background information on Amy.

While it is commonly assumed that most therapists have a small elderly clientele, reasons for this vary. One obvious factor may be that counselors are uncomfortable with this age group. Whether this is a conscious choice or one arising from unresolved problems, this choice should be respected. However, if one chooses to work with the older adult, I can safely say, with 25 years of experience, that the gains far outweigh the losses. Learning, modeling, and offering help and sustenance to our own future aging selves as represented by our clients is a joyous experience. A challenging and sometimes difficult road, it is a path most certainly worthwhile once undertaken.

Finally and in conclusion, Frank and Amy have, most concretely, "renewed" their marriage, if on another level. Love, of an abstract nature, has become that which is practiced in everyday life. Amy's love is less demanding and while still unable to express this, she shows it by her willingness to allow Frank his freedoms. Fears and anxieties have loosened their stranglehold on her, her life-force energy is now channeled toward that which she still enjoys, permitting others, and not only Frank, to be her companions.

Frank, keenly accepting of his role as caring husband, is able to live an independent existence away from Amy, immersed in his own activities and joys while also offering support to her. No longer trapped exclusively in their own scenarios, each can give the love to the other which first brought them together, if in a revised and modified form. As for me, still more was learned of life's strange and precious offerings by working with them. Although treatment, which lasted a little over a year, has since ended, the lessons learned by the three of us will go on and on for many years.

References

Aronson, M. (Ed.). (1988). *Alzheimer's disease and related disorders.* New York: Scribner.

Doty, P. (1986). Family care of the elderly: The role of public policy. *Milbank Quarterly, 64*(1), 34–75.

Ferraro, K. F. (Ed.). (1990). *Gerontology: Perspectives and issues.* New York: Springer.

Horowitz, A. (1985). Family caregiving to the frail elderly. In C. Eisendorfer (Ed.), *Annual review of gerontology and geriatrics.* (Vol. V, pp. 194–246). New York: Springer.

Muslin, H. L. (1992). *The psychotherapy of the elderly self.* New York: Brunner/Mazel.

Nemiroff, R. A., & Colarusso, C. A. (Eds.). (1994). *New dimensions in adult development.* New York: Basic Books.

Powell, L. (1993). *Alzheimer's disease.* New York: Addison-Wesley.

Sadavoy, J., Lazarus, L. W., & Jarvik, L. F. (1992). *Comprehensive review of geriatric psychiatry.* New York: American Association of Geriatric Psychiatry.

Stone, R., Cafferata, G. L., & Sangi, T. (1987). Caregivers of the frail elderly. *The Gerontologist, 27*, 616–626.

Viney, L. L. (1993). *Life stories.* New York: Wiley.

Weiner, M. B., Brok, A. J., & Snadowsky, A. M. (1987). *Working with the aged.* Norwalk, CT: Appleton-Century-Crofts.

Weiner, M. B., Teresi, J., & Streich, C. (1983). *Old people are a burden but not my parents.* New York: Prentice Hall.

White, M., & Weiner, M. B. (1986). *The theory and practice of self psychology.* New York: Brunner/Mazel.

■ ■ ■

11

Placement of the Elderly Parent in a Residential Health Care Facility: Impact on the Family

Shura Saul, EdD, BCD CSW

A residential health care facility, commonly known as a nursing home, is a place that serves and cares for physically and mentally dependent individuals (usually elderly) who require nursing and medical care that is not available in the home. Rehabilitative and related services of daily living accompany the basic nursing care. Because placement in such a facility usually occurs when family members are unable to provide needed care, the nursing home is also a family service agency—a role not commonly perceived.

A nursing home is a community of diverse residents and staff with a wide range of differing backgrounds—ethnic, cultural, economic, religious. These people all live and work together in a single facility because of a common need for nursing and medical care and related services. Their families are similarly diverse (Tepper, 1994) and so, too, are there diverse responses by family members to this challenging situation. Even within the relatively few nursing homes that serve homogeneous ethnic groups, there is diversity of family patterns and relationships. Yet some commonalities are identifiable (Hartford & Parsons, 1983).

Two pervasive stereotypes regarding nursing homes exercise a profoundly negative influence on the public mind. The first is the frightening and repugnant image of a nursing home as uncaring, hostile, or even brutal; an image that repels the healthier family members. This view may be reinforced by media exposés that tend to focus on the negative aspects of placement and not on the positive ones. The second is an equally destructive notion that families who place their elders in nursing homes do not care and prefer to abandon them. Both notions haunt and intimidate family members, some of whom may have harbored similar concepts for years but now find themselves and their elders in a desperate position. Both stereotypes interfere with a family's ability to anticipate or consider the realistic possibility that some day placement may become the only viable alternative for their elderly relative. When this eventuality occurs, a gamut of emotions is triggered within the family at the same time the dependent elder is grappling with massive changes in his or her own life.

Placement of an elder in a health care facility is a point of sharp discontinuity for both the elder and the family, causing significant intrapsychic and interpersonal distress for all concerned. Even in those situations where placement offers relief and the promise of improved care to the family and older person, both may experience a sense of loss, of failure, of self reproach. It therefore becomes very important for counselors to maintain, support, and encourage positive and appropriate family relationships. Such efforts benefit the older person, the family members, and the facility and caregiving staff as well. Reparative efforts must consider the attitudes, needs, feelings, and circumstances of those three groups and the related cluster of their problems. Professional interventions addressing these sensitive problems must recognize that this is a period of profound pain for all concerned. Understanding and support for both residents and family members can be developed through individual and group counseling, case conferences, family counseling, and the maintenance of open communication between administration, staff, family, and resident.

Of primary consideration for the counselor are the feelings of the older person, which encompass the following:

1. affective responses to a succession of losses associated with aging and chronic illness and to the succession of incidents experienced prior to placement and during the admission process;
2. response to the specific physical or emotional illness that precipitated placement;

3. emotional and physical adaptive responses to the trauma and demands of the changes (e.g., losses of home, privacy, and control over one's daily life, assault on identity, and strain on all coping capacities);
4. adaptive responses to the immediate circumstances of the communal living situation;
5. inner conflict regarding possible changes in family relationships and roles; and
6. pervasive, underlying fear of the imminence of death.

At this point, the older person has experienced rejection, change, and threatening discontinuities in life; has been physically and emotionally assaulted; is exhausted and possibly bewildered. Feelings combine anger, frustration, impotence, and fear. The person may be confused and disoriented, may suffer memory loss, and may be in a mild to severe state of shock. Feelings toward the family reflect this range of emotions. The older person may be angry at, ashamed of, defensive about, loving toward, dependent on, and rejecting of the family—all at the same time!

The feelings and attitudes of family members mirror those of the older person. They may be concerned with any or all of the following:

1. distress over the conflict between the needs of the older and younger family members; such conflicts have usually been a burden to the middle generation who may be torn between conflicting economic, psychological, physical, and social needs of younger family members and by too many management demands in use of time, space, chores, and money in the routines of daily living (Blenkner, 1965);
2. affective responses to earlier or ongoing conflicts or problems in their relationships with the older person;
3. despair over losses suffered by the older person;
4. despair over loss of control of the caring situation; feelings of inadequacy related to care of spouse or parent; loss of one's own caring role; and
5. fear of death—ultimate and irreversible separation from spouse or parent figure.

The Admission Process

Admission to a nursing home is a crisis situation, the specifics of which are often beyond the family's control. Usually the older person is passive and ill, so that the family is forced to take an active role in decision making. This fact alone tends to heighten the emotional reactions of both family and older person. These may include guilt, sorrow, grief, anger, frustration, relief, a sense of failure, and fear. These feelings may be consciously recognized or denied, but the common denominator is the same. They reflect distress, ambivalence, and confusion over the act of placement (Sutker, 1993).

The change from living in one's own home to the nursing home is usually triggered by one of two possible traumas. The older person may have been hospitalized, often after a traumatic physical event such as heart attack, fracture, or stroke. The other possibility is that placement is arranged while the older person is still living at home. This decision is usually made due to a disintegrating home situation in which the increasing dependency needs of the elder are paralleled by the decreasing ability of the family to meet these needs. Such a situation culminates in the recognition that placement in a nursing home has become the only solution to a difficult situation.

Regardless of which of these paths has led to the nursing home, this change is experienced as a trauma by both the older person and the family.

> Most families have two obstacles to hurdle prior to accepting a nursing home solution; they must overcome their own aversion and the opposition of the potential nursing home resident. It is hard to pinpoint the exact moment when institutionalization becomes a necessary move—what provides the tipping point forcing the decision. ...But for most families, whenever the tipping point comes...it is a painful finality in terms of their parents' lives. (Silverstone & Hyman, 1982, p. 206)

For most families, as well as for the elderly resident, placement signifies a sharp change in the family constellation and in the organization of family life. Whether or not the home care situation had been long-lived, and even regardless of the quality of intrafamilial relationships, the actual act of placement is difficult both to contemplate and to enact.

Most families are quite unprepared to cope with the world of residential health care. They are generally not well informed about nursing homes, long-term care, and the process of placement. They are also largely ignorant and distressed about such details as finances, life in the nursing home, and their own relationship to the long-term care system. Finally, they are confused by the complexities of the change, by the new circumstances of the life of the older person, by the demands of their own new roles and relationships, and by the conflicting and generally distressing range of emotions that beset them.

Impact on Family Members

The depth and power of the family's emotions, while different both between and among different families, require both empathy and understanding. Placement of an elderly family member may have different consequences for various members of the family (e.g., spouses, adult children, grandchildren, elderly siblings, extended family). The sharp and painful changes in the older person's circumstances of dependency, physical decline, psychological and emotional state, status, and living condition create distress in other family members. For some there may also be the fear that this might portend their own future.

Spouses

Probably the most severely affected person in the family is the husband or wife of the resident. The spouse who remains at home experiences a radical change in his or her own lifestyle. No matter how arduous the home care situation might have been, or even how unexpected the relief of placement might be, the spouse now remains living alone. This new situation requires coping with the concrete realities of the "single" life while still maintaining a relationship with the marital partner. The spouse is deprived of a social and sexual partner, and his or her affectional needs are often frustrated. Solitary meals, lonely days and nights, changes in financial and social situations, the need to visit the nursing home and cope with its pressures, and the altered pattern and quality of the marital relationship are all part of a severely altered existence. These concrete realities are accompanied by profound feelings of loss, a sense of failure, frustration, and remorse related to the spouse's role in the placement process, anger at the unfairness of this unexpected turn in senescence, and disquieting questions about one's own future.

Elderly Siblings

Some siblings have been sharing a home and are now faced with a situation similar to that of a spouse. Often siblings who remain at home have been coping with their own changes in health and social relationships at the same time that they have been caring for the more needy sister or brother. The placement process is almost as bewildering and threatening to a sibling as it is to a spouse. Elderly sisters or brothers, themselves single, may need help in adapting to the changes in their own circumstances that accompany the placement of their sibling.

Siblings who have not been living with the ailing brother or sister are also affected in various ways that might include assuming new responsibilities for the resident (e.g., helping with finances, shopping, visiting). They, too, may respond with a range of emotions to the placement including concern over the sibling's dependency and loss of control, concern for their own future, and feelings of remorse over earlier problems in the relationship.

Adult Children

There is no single word to describe the first generation offspring of an older person. (At the time of placement, these people might themselves be grandparents.) The term *adult offspring* barely reflects the important family bond it represents. The term *adult child* is almost an oxymoron, yet it does speak to the crux of this emotional relationship. It suggests the duality of feelings and relationships that surface when a parent becomes dependent on the child, especially when the "child" may also be aging.

> When nursing home placement is necessary for an elderly parent, realistic sons and daughters must face an imperfect situation and at the same time face two other painful realities: the irreversible deterioration of a person they love, and their own inability or unwillingness to care for that person. (Silverstone & Hyman, 1982, p. 205)

One's parent is the authority figure of earliest memory; the person who represents (in whatever idiosyncratic way) adulthood; the person who first linked the child to family, society, and future; the one who taught values; the one through whom superego and social conscience were shaped; the one from whom the child first learned love, hate, and all the emotions that propel us through the Scylla and Charybdis of life.

The bonds between parent and child, forged during the years of childhood, adulthood, and senescence, may have been strengthened or weakened by the specific vicissitudes of the family's life. A range of emotional ties, some clear, some confused, has developed. The significance of the parent–child relationship is pervasive even when the outward behavior of either or both may seem to suggest otherwise. Actions and reactions of adult children will vary with the family history and the family secrets, with the personalities of the individuals involved, and with the specific circumstances of each. This is nowhere clearer than when a parent enters a nursing home (Greene, 1986).

Different Ways of Caring

The negative stereotypes of family are shattered when the behavior of family members is observed and understood. Some people seem to take placement in their stride, cope with the psychic pain, and adapt to the change. They may assume new responsibility, visit regularly, bring appropriate gifts, and take part in the new life of the parent. Others may stay away, generally because they are either unable or unwilling to face the parent or the environment. Still others may maintain "long distance" connections through mail or telephone calls. On the surface, feelings and relationships may appear obvious, cut and dried (Saul, 1973).

However, some of the following examples suggest the need for a deeper, more empathic look. Consider the anxious daughters of Mrs. Sackson, who weeps quietly at each visit; Mrs. Wright's angry son who scolds her loudly but comes weekly to take her on outings; the tormented college professor son of Mrs. Jones who does not come at all but whose wife visits every Monday afternoon; Mrs. Harris's children who lied, denying that she had ever been in a mental hospital for fear she'd be labeled "crazy"; the conflicted young daughters of Mrs. Kane asking the hospital discharge coordinator, "Shouldn't we wait another month before we 'put her in?'" There is the daughter who finds fault with everything that is done for her mother. There are the daughters who visit, bring clothing, and talk to the doctors but never show any emotion or sign of affection toward their mother. There are the adult children who never come, never call. These are all different ways of expressing inadequacy in the face of these massive parental needs.

The various expressions of emotional behavior (overanxiety, rejecting behavior, indifference) are, for the most part, signs of some level of caring within a chaotic, anxious time of crisis and bewilderment. All may be viewed as responses to the pressures of the change.

Interventions: The Family Counselor

Counseling interventions to help family members during this difficult time are based on several underlying concepts:

1. There must be a basic belief in and respect for the family bond, no matter how damaged it appears. This suggests the need for adopting a nonjudgmental stance toward both family members and the resident.
2. There should be no attempt to repair damaged relationships that developed in earlier times. The goal is not for family members to "kiss and make-up" but to develop a pattern of interaction between the family members and the person in the nursing home.
3. Family history and secrets are acknowledged. Where they have become impediments to a reasonable current relationship they may be dealt with, sensitively and appropriately, with the clear goal of establishing an appropriate pattern of relationship. Mr. G., a "sweet old man," was constantly calling for his son who "only visits once a week." The social worker asked to see the son, explaining his father's complaint. Although he had not been asked for intimate details, the son launched into a description of horrendous family abuse by the father. It was clear that this son was fulfilling his filial duty by visiting once a week and that was all he could be expected to do.

For the most part, all family members (especially spouses and adult children) may be helped through some type of counseling. This may be offered by a staff member of the care facility (e.g., social worker, nurse, therapist) or by a family counselor. Family counselors can assist in the following tasks:

1. They can clarify the resident's feelings about placement and ease the burden of negative feelings (such as guilt, despair, shame).
2. They can help the family members recognize and accept (a) the validity of the placement, (b) their own feelings regarding this placement, and (c) the feelings of the older relative. For the family member who complains constantly about treatment of the resident, it is important to establish the facts and to make whatever corrections are possible. The relative may also be involved in developing appropriate solutions to real situations. Complaints must be understood within the framework

of frustration and helplessness that family members may be feeling. Support may be given by suggesting that "No one can love your mother (or wife, father, etc.) the way you do...no one can give the care you have given...but an effort is being made and you can still participate in your relative's care and life."

3. They can free family members to maintain a continuity of relationship with the resident through appropriate roles and activities in the new living situation. Visiting may be difficult for family members who find it hard to see their relative in this environment, or to tolerate it themselves. A relative may find visiting awkward, not knowing what to do or say. This situation may be eased through suggesting pleasant, appropriate activities such as sharing an appropriate project with the relative, reading together, developing a family tree, talking about old times, creating a family picture album, or playing a game of cards, checkers, or chess. Family members may be invited to accompany the relative to suitable group activities, thus helping to link the resident with the life in the facility.

4. They can help the family member become an appropriate link in the chain of caring for the relative.

   Mrs. L.'s daughter, a widow age 74 herself, visited her mother twice a week. Each time, she found some fault with the care given to her mother. She became known to the staff as "the pest." At a conference with her, the staff learned that Mrs. L. was her daughter's sole remaining relative, that she had been caring for her mother for many years, and had found it difficult to relinquish her role. The daughter was invited to attend the care plan meetings and participate in suggestions for mother's care. After several counseling sessions she was helped to find ways to continue her role, for example, by accompanying her mother to activities and participating appropriately in her mother's care and life.

5. They can show understanding, appreciation of, and empathy for the specific circumstances, problems, and needs of some family members.

   Mrs. A. (daughter of an 86-year-old resident in the nursing home) visited weekly. She was consistently berated by her mother for not visiting more often. Her visits became less frequent and briefer and she finally confessed to the counselor that she found it very difficult to visit at all. During the conference, she explained that her 10-year old son was a handicapped child with special needs and that she was also caring for a frail father-in-law who lived with her family. In addition, her mother-in-law, placed in another facility, was in a late stage of Alzheimer's disease. Obviously, it was important to empathize with these problems to help her be comfortable in doing as much or as little as she could for her mother. With such support, her visits became less stressful and more satisfying to mother and daughter.

6. They can suggest creative solutions for communication and connectedness.

Mrs. F., a daughter-in-law, revealed that her husband went into a serious depression after every visit to his mother. He stopped visiting on the advice of his psychiatrist but felt very upset at severing connections with his mother. It was suggested that he write her a note instead and that she would be helped to respond. This proved to be helpful to all.

Mrs. G., a daughter who lived out of town and could only visit every other week was helped to arrange a daily morning telephone call to her mother. Mother would be wheeled to the telephone at the appointed time and both enjoyed a daily chat with little or no stress. Mother's day was enhanced and daughter's feelings relieved.

Family Support Groups

Participation in a family support group can be very useful in helping families to cope with their feelings. The value of groups for helping people cope with emotional stress has been summarized in Yalom's listing of the "curative factors" of group therapy. Among these he identified the instillation of hope, universality, imparting of information, development of socializing techniques, and interpersonal learning (Yalom, 1975). All of these factors are addressed by participation in family support groups. Family members enter the world of the nursing home feeling isolated and assaulted by events beyond their control. Sharing their experiences with others "in the same boat" helps them to cope with the difficult present situation.

Two types of group experiences are generally available: the family council within the facility and a therapeutic support group either in the facility or elsewhere in the community (e.g., a mental health center).

For some family members, family councils provide information, education, and involvement in the practical aspects of care that help to ease emotional strain and make placement more acceptable. Family councils can offer a range of activities that help family members to feel part of their relative's world and to play a significant role in their relative's life. Family council meetings can bring relatives and residents together with administrative and staff leadership to clarify general concerns, policies, and practices of the home.

For other family members, a therapeutic support group may be more helpful. This group is geared more directly to the emotional concerns of those who are willing to participate. It is generally a smaller, more intimate group where feelings may be eased through the exploration of common experiences related to the unique circumstances of the members (Butler, Lewis, & Sunderland, 1991).

Separate groups for spouses, whose problems and concerns differ somewhat from those of adult children, have proven to be useful. The advantages of such a group include the opportunities for participants to share experiences, suggestions, and ideas that might ease their common suffering; to feel less alone and isolated in their plight; and to experience group (and leader) support in their daily struggles to cope with their concerns about their spouses and themselves. Adult children may find participation in similar groups worthwhile. Stress on the family as a unit can be helped through family counseling by a family therapist.

Exceptional Situations

Two circumstances that exacerbate family distress and require family counseling involve the elder who suffers from some form of dementia and the elder who is terminally ill. Both of these situations demand special sensitivity, knowledge, and skill on the part of the counselor.

Dementia

It is extremely painful for family members to cope with their own feelings about the relative suffering from some form of dementia. In the case of patients suffering from Alzheimer's disease, families experience extreme despair and feelings of loss. As one daughter said, "My mother died some years ago. Yet this is still my mother."

> Unrealistic family expectations can compound problems arising from a patient's altered character. It is very difficult...for close kin to appreciate the changes a brain impaired person has undergone. Misinterpretation of the patient's behavioral deterioration often complicates...problems for family members....Most family members...suffer from depression. (Lindeman, 1984, pp. 13–14)

Family members of these patients need special attention and may find a support group helpful. In addition to the previously mentioned values of a support group, a group led by a leader with expertise in dementia can help family members understand and cope with the personality changes and the loss of cognition in their relative. Spouses or adult children can be aided in accepting the patient's general deterioration, bizarre and unexpected behavior, and altered means of communication.

Terminal Illness

The grieving and anticipation of loss for the family members of the terminally ill patient can be very severe. They may experience a range of emotions such as fear, anger, denial, or an inability to express their feelings. There may be "unfinished emotional business" between the patient and family members that may interfere with compassionate and satisfying visiting. The sensitivity of the counselor is very important as opportunities for closure in the relationship decrease. All efforts should be directed at creating opportunities for satisfying visits. Some people need to have control of many details of the patient's life and care. Others may want all possible information. Still others may require just the opposite. The empathic, understanding, nonjudgmental stance of the helping person is vital in maintaining the fragile relationship between patient and family member. Spouses, adult children, and other family members must be helped to retain the most possible satisfying relationship with the patient, so that the impending death will inflict the least amount of guilt, invoke the least amount of anger. Death must be viewed as a merciful release from pain and suffering.

When the patient dies, continuity of support should be maintained, if only briefly, through the process and procedures following death. Bereavement counseling may or may not be appropriate, depending on the individuals involved. It is universally appropriate, however, to express caring concern for the family and to cooperate in a helpful way in the aftermath of the loss.

Summary

When the chronically ill, dependent resident of a nursing home is viewed as a whole person who has lived a long and unique life before becoming a resident, it becomes clear that his or her family remains involved in the altered life situation. Family members need assistance in adapting to this change. Family counseling should include information, education, emotional support, and opportunities for the continuity or restoration of healthy relationships. Caring and compassion for residents and their families are key elements in the process.

References

Blenkner, M. (1965). Social work and family relationships in later life with some thoughts on filial maturity. In E. Shanas & G. F. Streit (Eds.), *Social structure and the family: Generational relationships* (pp. 46–59). Englewood Cliffs, NJ: Prentice Hall.

Butler, R., Lewis, M., & Sunderland, T. (1991). *Aging and mental health* (4th ed.). New York: Macmillan.

Greene, R. R. (1986). *Social work with the aged and their families*. New York: Aldine de Gruyter.

Hartford, M. E., & Parsons, R. (1983). Uses of groups with relatives of dependent older adults. In S. Saul (Ed.), *Group work with the frail elderly* (pp. 77-89). New York: Haworth Press.

Lindeman, D. (1984). The psychosocial aspects of Alzheimer's disease. In U. S. Department of Health and Human Services, *Alzheimer's disease handbook* (Vol. I, pp. 13–14). DHHS Publication No. (OHDS) 84-20813.

Saul, S. (1973). *Aging: An album of people growing old*. New York: Wiley.

Silverstone, B., & Hyman, H. K. (1982). *You and your aging parents*. New York: Pantheon Books.

Sutker, R. K. (1993). Is the nursing home right for you? In J. A. Toner, L. M. Tepper, & B. Greenfield (Eds.), *Long term care* (pp. 80–87). Philadelphia: Charles Press.

Tepper, L. (1994). Family relationships in later life. In I. Gutheil (Ed.), *Work with older people* (pp. 422–461). New York: Fordham University Press.

Yalom, I. D. (1975). *The theory and practice of group psychotherapy*. New York: Basic Books.

■ ■ ■

12

The Effect of Parental Illness and Loss on Adult Children

Kenneth J. Doka, PhD

O f all family crises, few are as wrenching as the illness and death of an aging parent. The event is a developmental mark that can radically change not only the lives of all family members, but also the dynamics of relationships through the extended family. It is wrought with emotional turmoil, cognitive distress, and behavioral disturbance.

This chapter considers the effect of the illness and death of an aging parent on surviving members of the family. It begins by reviewing the effect of parental aging, fragility, and illness on the development of the adult child. Next, the issues and stresses that arise as these adult children cope with the illness and death of that aging parent are considered. Finally, there is a discussion of practical interventions that caregivers may use as they assist individuals and families in coping with that crisis.

I must begin with a caveat. By its very nature a chapter of this type must be general. Families, though, are not. They are defined by their own dynamics, histories, and myths. Families are influenced by their social classes, cultural customs, and religious beliefs. They have their own distinct patterns, roles, and relationships. In addition, each illness creates its own distinct issues for each member.

The Aging of Parents: A Developmental Perspective

The aging of parents seems to have a strong developmental effect on their adult children. Blenkner (1965), for example, proposed that the aging and subsequent decline of a parent creates a new sense of "filial maturity" toward the offspring. Usually this begins with a "filial crisis" where the adult children are forced to recognize that their parents have aged and are now frail. The adult children recognize that the parents are no longer the awesome or awful mythical beings of childhood on whom one could always depend. The children begin to see the parents as real people with real needs. The adult children also realize that they may be called to become caregivers for their parents. To Blenkner (1965), filial maturity means that adult children need to realistically acknowledge their parents' frailty and become willing to take a supportive role in their parents' lives.

This new relationship can be difficult to achieve. The aging of a parent can be exceedingly threatening to a child. Doka (1989) proposed that one of the key developmental issues that adults must struggle with in midlife is their own awareness of mortality. Middle-aged adults recognize that they are mortal. The aging and death of a parent is one factor that may cause midlife adults to confront their own personal mortality. As long as parents are alive, they act as a buffer against death. The adult child can still feel a generation from death. The dying older parent then may become a personal harbinger to the adult children of their own eventual aging and death.

In addition, the new relationship that is forged as parents age may also create strong ambivalence. Parents, while grateful for the support of their children, may resent their dependency on their children and the intrusion of the children on their autonomy. Adult children may be pleased they can be supportive but also resent the new responsibilities and demands.

Not only are these relationships ambivalent, they are often unstable. Every new crisis, each subsequent parental decline or recovery will continue to cause changes in the pattern of interaction.

Despite these struggles, parent–child relationships tend to remain strong. Bengston, Olander, and Haddad (1976) used the concept of *developmental stakes* to explain the durable nature of parent–child relationships. They maintained that the relationship is important developmentally for each person. Adult children provide a sense of "symbolic immortality" that sustains them as they face death. Parents can derive comfort from having raised responsible children who will perpetuate their memory. For adult children, the assumption of care of an older parent becomes a responsibility. These developmental stakes of comfort and care hold relationships intact against the threatening forces of later-life crisis.

The Illness of an Elderly Parent

A parent's life-threatening illness is one of the most difficult crises that an adult child faces. Many chronic diseases increasingly have become amenable to medical treatment. As a result, many older persons may live a considerable period of time while they struggle with life-threatening illness.

Life-threatening illness may be viewed as a series of phases, each with its own problems and issues for effective coping (Doka, 1993). Each phase will raise different concerns not only for the aging parents but also for their adult children.

The earliest phase occurs before the diagnosis. In this prediagnostic period, the elderly parent may be struggling with symptoms. Often persons delay seeking medical treatment while they watch the symptom, self-medicate, or seek the advice of family and friends. Elderly persons are particularly likely to delay treatment, perhaps believing that the symptoms are typical of the aches and pains experienced within the aging process. When they finally do seek medical treatment, the delay may have negatively affected their medical options and survival (Doka, 1993).

It is often worthwhile to explore this period with families. Prediagnostic behaviors may indicate basic coping strategies, fears and anxieties, and social support. It is important to assess individual actions as well as relationship dynamics. Did children encourage a doctor's visit? Was the elderly parent reticent about sharing concerns? Did one spouse attempt to use the adult children to force a course of action?

The second phase is the diagnostic phase. The time when a life-threatening illness is diagnosed is often a period of acute crisis, in some cases, nearly as difficult as death itself. Diagnosis usually takes place over a period of weeks as various tests are completed. This period usually is a time of both intense affect and interaction between parents and children.

The chronic phase is the period when parents and their families have to cope with the realities of treatment. While the sense of urgency generally recedes, there is a constant struggle to live day by day, coping with both the demands of daily life and the effects of the illness and the treatment. All the demands of care—financial, emotional, and physical—can stress family resources. Depending on the illness, the chronic phase can be of varying duration. In some cases, such as multiple sclerosis, the period can last indefinitely.

Some persons may recover. Even in these cases the illness may have residual effects throughout the family system. The illness is likely to have generated new patterns of interaction that may need to be renegotiated after recovery. For example, the parent may have become dependent on the adult child and, even in the absence of illness, continue that dependence. Or the adult child may find it difficult to relinquish the roles he or she played during the parent's illness. In any case, the pattern of parent–adult child interaction is unlikely to automatically revert to the previous pattern.

In other cases, a person may move into a terminal phase. Here the individual and family prepare for death. This approaching encounter with death may intensify both caregiving demands on the adult child and the emotional tone between parents and children.

Throughout the course of a parent's life-threatening illness, the adult child has a twofold task. First, he or she may need to support the ill parent. The adult child may be called on to shepherd the parent to hospitals and doctors, to negotiate with caregivers, and to assist with treatment. The parent's illness may mean that the adult child may have to take an increasing role in managing the parent's household.

Second, in addition to supporting the ill parent, the adult child may need to support the other parent. That parent may need emotional support as he or she copes with crises of a spouse's illness and his or her own anticipatory grief. Often the illness of one parent may affect the other parent's well-being, health, or survival. For example, one spouse may be providing critical care or support for his or her mate as they both struggle with increasing frailty. When one person becomes ill, the other's health may be threatened.

As mentioned earlier, the adult child's increasing involvement in the lives of older parents is fraught with the potential for conflict. Often parents and children will have great ambivalence as they struggle together with issues of autonomy and dependency. In other cases, though, parents and their adult children may have positive experiences. Adult children have the opportunity to affirm their parents' roles in their lives and finish business, for example, exchange validation, extend forgiveness, or provide a sense of closure (Doka, 1993). In addition, this new role can contribute to the adult child's sense of responsibility, raising self-esteem and conveying to the older parents a sense that they were successful in the parental role (Bengston, Olander, & Haddad, 1976).

Life-threatening illness then is inevitably a family illness. The illness of an elderly parent will affect everyone within the family system. The adult children may differ in their coping styles. They may resent differing levels of involvement and responsibility of other siblings. In addition, the spouse and children of the adult child may resent the attention paid to the ill parent (Doka, 1993).

Conflicts between family members are not unusual. These conflicts may be of three types. First, there are continuing conflicts. Such conflicts have a long history. Here the illness and the problems caused by it simply become an arena for continuing long-lasting fights. For example, in one case a brother and sister were in constant conflict over whether or not an ill parent should be institutionalized. This argument was just part of a long series of conflicts that had begun in early childhood.

In other cases, the illness may reactivate conflicts that had been dormant. For example, in one case, the illness of a parent reactivated a daughter's feelings of resentment based on her perception that her parents always favored her brother. Though she had become the major caregiver, her parents always seemed to comment on the support that the brother provided, reviving her earlier feelings surrounding favoritism. Similarly, in another case, a wife's attention to her parents during illness reactivated her husband's feeling that his wife placed her parents before him.

Conflicts also can be new. The tension of life-threatening illness can raise new issues and concerns for families. In one family, for example, there was considerable tension between previously close sisters over whether or not they should sign a "do not resuscitate" directive.

The illness of the parent has a strong effect on the adult children. They may be coping with the new demands posed by the illness as well as with their own emotions and anticipatory grief. The adult child begins to grieve both the potential loss of a parent as well as all the losses that may have been experienced at that point in the illness (e.g., loss of mobility and freedom due to caregiving demands, loss of mutually pleasurable activities for parent and adult child) (Rando, 1988). The illness of a parent may challenge the child's sense of mortality. The adult child may have strong feelings of countertransference, seeing their own responses to illness and death in the ways parents cope. Their sense of self may be threatened when a parent dies, for a part of one's own past may seem to die as well.

In summary, the life-threatening illness of a parent has profound effects throughout the family system. Counselors can help by having members explore the particular issues that arise at each phase of the illness, by validating the emotional responses of the members of the family system, by assisting them in examining and understanding the ways that each member of the system copes, and by helping them in comprehending and resolving conflicts. This may involve exploring the relationship between the adult child and aging parent because the sense of caregiving burden is influenced by the role the parent played throughout the life of the child. When that role is perceived as positive, the sense of subjective or felt burden is mitigated. When the parent's role is largely negative, adult children may perceive even minimal caregiving demands as highly intrusive (Dwyer, Lee, & Jankowski, 1994).

The Death of an Older Parent

The death of an aging parent has substantial effects on survivors. Spouses, of course, are particularly vulnerable. The literature has identified that older widows may have a very different bereavement experience than younger widows (Parkes, 1972; Sanders, 1980). Older widowed spouses may have certain supports not as readily available to younger widows. For example, older widows and widowers may find many widowed peers, providing a natural circle of support. In addition, prior loss experiences may make the experiences of grief less strange. Although the experience of loss is traumatic, it is also normative; that is, many older widows and widowers recognize their own and their spouses' fragility and finitude. Death, even when sudden, may not seem like a complete surprise.

Even though older widows and widowers may have certain supports, they also experience unique difficulties. Older persons often face multiple losses within a short space of time. They cope not only with one loss but rather a series of losses.

The death of a spouse can also have a negative effect on the mental and physical health of the surviving spouse (Parkes, 1972). In fact, older spouses experience higher rates of mortality within the years following the loss (Raphael, 1983). One reason for this might be that the death of a spouse may adversely affect the lifestyle practices of the survivor. For instance, the death of a spouse may influence the survivor's diet and eating habits, exercise patterns, adherence to a medical regimen, or their ability to function within the home environment. It is critical for counselors to explore these issues with surviving spouses.

The death of an older adult affects not only the spouse. Adult children can experience a profound sense of loss. They may mourn the loss of a unique and longstanding role in their own lives, one at least ideally based on unconditional love and acceptance (Rando, 1988; Sanders, 1989). The loss of parents may mean a loss of the ties to childhood and one's past. It also may leave unfinished business such as the opportunity to see a child become successful or share in grandchildren (Moss & Moss, 1989; Rando, 1988). It may remind surviving children of their own mortality (Doka, 1989) and provide a developmental push, forcing adult children into new roles and responsibilities (Osterweis, Solomen, & Green, 1984). It may create profound changes in relationships with siblings now that a parental focal point is missing. In some cases, usually those with preexisting conflicts, debate over inheritance can create considerable rancor among surviving siblings (Doka, 1992). Even in the absence of conflicts, the death of a parent can create additional losses as siblings sell a family home or divide possessions (Doka, 1992).

The loss of an older parent can be complicated if others discount that loss. As Moss and Moss (1989) indicated, the grief for an older parent can be disenfranchised by others. While everyone recognizes the grief of a 12-year-old who has lost his or her parents, the grief of a 42-year-old adult orphan may not be validated by others. Though adult children experience a deep sense of loss, they may be led to feel that they have no socially recognized right to grieve when others define the death as normative or even merciful.

Counselors can be very helpful in validating the normalcy of grief, exploring the variety of losses a person experiences with the death of a parent, and helping to identify times when feelings of loss may be accentuated such as anniversary reactions, significant life events (e.g., the birth of a new child), or settlement reactions (e.g., receiving insurance money, selling the parental home).

Implications for Family Counselors

The illness or death of an older parent is a significant developmental event for adult children. The role of a counselor in this situation is similar to any other crisis—to enable persons to use their own coping styles and resourses to surmount the crisis. Counselors can have a significant role in validating and exploring the feelings and reactions of affected individuals and family systems (Herr & Weakland, 1979).

In assisting families, counselors may find an approach called "network intervention" useful in mobilizing family systems. Originally developed to help troubled children deal with emotional crises, it can be applied to a wide variety of crisis situations (Thorman, 1982). In this approach, a network of family and friends is invited to meet in the home of the bereaved person for a period of two days for 6 to 8 hours each day to solve a particular problem. This approach is effective when there is a clearly defined problem, an established network willing to assist, and a family open to share the problem and options for a solution within a larger setting. For example, it could be an extremely useful technique if a family is called on to provide physical care and assistance to an ill parent for a period of time that taxes the resources of any given family member.

Network intervention is only one example of techniques that counselors may use to help families meet the crisis of an older parent's illness or death. No matter what approach is used, the counselor's role is best perceived as an adjunct, assisting and enabling families to find and achieve their own resolutions. Effective counselors act as guides and advisors.

However painful or difficult, the illness and death of aging parents is a normal part of an adult's development. How adult children resolve these crises may be critical in developing coping mechanisms that will allow them to effectively and eventually face the crises of their own life-threatening illness and death.

References

Bengston, V., Olander, G., & Haddad, A. (1976). The generation gap and aging family members: Toward a conceptual model. In J. Gubrium (Ed.), *Time, roles and self in old age* (pp. 237–263). New York: Human Services Press.

Blenkner, M. (1965). Social work and family relationships in later life with some thoughts on filial maturity. In G. Shanas and G. Streib (Eds.), *Social structure and the family* (pp. 46–61). Englewood Cliffs, NJ: Prentice Hall.

Doka, K. J. (1989). The awareness of mortality in midlife: Implications for later life. *Gerontology Review, 2,* 19–28.

Doka, K. J. (1992). The monkey's paw: The role of inheritance in the resolution of grief. *Death Studies, 16,* 45–58.

Doka, K. J. (1993). *Living with life threatening illness: A guide for individuals, families and caregivers.* Lexington, MA: Lexington Press.

Dwyer, J. W., Lee, G. R., & Jankowski, T. B. (1994). Reciprocity, elder satisfaction, and caregiver stress and burden: The exchange of aid in the family caregiving relationship. *Journal of Marriage and the Family, 56,* 35–43.

Herr, J., & Weakland, J. (1979). *Counseling elders and their families.* New York: Springer.

Moss, M., & Moss, S. (1989). Death of the very old. In K. Doka (Ed.), *Disenfranchised grief: Recognizing hidden sorrow* (pp. 213–228). Lexington, MA: Lexington Books.

Osterweis, M., Solomen, S., & Green, M. (Eds.). (1984). *Bereavement: Reactions, consequences and care.* Washington, DC: National Academy Press.

Parkes, C. M. (1972). *Bereavement: Studies of grief in adult life.* New York: International University Press.

Rando, T. A. (1988). *Grieving: How to go on living when someone you love dies.* Lexington, MA: Lexington Books.

Raphael, B. (1983). *The anatomy of bereavement.* New York: Basic Books.

Sanders, C. (1980). Comparison of younger and older spouses in bereavement outcome. *Omega, 11,* 217–237.

Sanders, C. (1989). *Grief: The mourning after.* New York: Wiley.

Thorman, G. (1982). *Helping troubled families: A social work perspective.* New York: Aldine.

■ ■ ■